AF700585

Awesome Women in Medicine—Book 2

20 Inspiring Stories of Those Who Made a Difference

Peggy Hadley
(Peggyhadley1008@gmail.com)

Boogie Publishing
(Boogiepublishing@gmail.com)

For Megan... the strongest one of us all.

A Note from the Author

I hope you enjoy *Awesome Women in Medicine* and all the books in the "Awesome Women" series. They were written to show girls and young women the power they truly do hold. If you're so inclined, please leave a review, and I would also love to hear from you at either of the email addresses below:

- Peggyhadley1008@gmail.com
- Boogiepublishing@gmail.com

Table of Contents

Introduction

Did you know that only 10% of medical degrees in the 1800s were awarded to women (Justin, n.d.)? Yet pioneers like Elizabeth Blackwell shattered this barrier, forging a path for future generations. Imagine standing at the doorway of a prestigious institution, gazing at a world that tells you it's not meant for you. For centuries, women with dreams of donning a white coat or wielding a stethoscope faced insurmountable odds. They were met with skepticism, rejection, and sometimes outright hostility. And yet, they persevered.

We're here to read about the women who didn't let anyone tell them what they could or couldn't be. Women like Mary Eliza Mahoney, the first African American woman to become a professional nurse, didn't just pursue personal dreams. Their true mission was to change the world for everyone. When you learn about these stories of audacity, you'll discover dreams are attainable, no matter the obstacles. These stories of perseverance are like binoculars that allow you to see beyond societal limitations.

These women's inspiring lives are bridges connecting the past to the present, helping us understand that each challenge overcome is a stepping stone to greater achievements. The struggles they faced aren't relics of times past; they resonate with the challenges young people encounter today. Whether it's being dismissed, underestimated, or stereotyped, the fight for recognition and equality continues.

The experiences of these women echo the very real challenges you might face in your pursuit of a career in medicine. This book aims to give you insights into how to build resilience and determination so you can stand confidently and leave your own indelible marks on history.

This book isn't just a collection of biographies; it's a call to action. It invites you to see these remarkable women not as distant figures in textbooks but as mentors and role models. Their stories are proof that you too can rise above the constraints society might place on you.

As you turn the pages, consider the possibility that the next great breakthrough in medicine could come from you. Visualize yourself in a lab coat, making discoveries that change lives. Imagine your name etched into the timeline of medical advancements, a testament to your hard work and dedication. The road ahead will have its challenges, but each step forward is a victory against those who've doubted you.

You are the future. You hold the potential to redefine what's possible in medicine and science. Just like Elizabeth, Mary, and many others, your contributions can shape the world, making it a better, more inclusive place. The stories within these pages are mirrors reflecting the potential within you—the potential to break barriers, innovate, and inspire future generations.

Let this book be your guide on a journey of empowerment and discovery. Let it remind you that, although the path may be difficult, the destination is worth every struggle. Embrace the power of knowledge, and begin with the understanding that you have the strength to overcome any obstacle, follow your passion, and make a difference.

So, are you ready to embark on a transformative journey? Are you prepared to take up the torch passed down by these incredible trailblazers? Let their legacies fuel your aspirations and energize your pursuits. Together, we'll explore the incredible impact of women in medicine and imagine the groundbreaking possibilities that await you.

Your story is yet to be written, your dreams are waiting to unfold, and your contribution to medicine is poised to leave a lasting legacy. Welcome to a world where anything is possible when you dare to dream big and strive for excellence.

Chapter 1:

Elizabeth Blackwell—A Pioneer in Medicine

Elizabeth Blackwell was one of the first female trailblazers in the field of medicine. At a time when the world viewed women's roles through the narrow lens of domesticity, Elizabeth envisioned something greater for herself and others. Her determination led her into uncharted territory, breaking barriers in an era filled with skepticism toward women in professional fields.

Elizabeth struggled against societal norms that sought to confine her to traditional roles and courageously applied to medical schools despite repeated rejections. The Geneva Medical College opened its doors to her under unique circumstances, and she faced uncountable trials while pursuing her degree. Alongside her academic success, you'll see the broader impact of her achievements, from establishing the New York Infirmary to inspiring future female physicians.

Overcoming Gender Barriers in Education

Elizabeth Blackwell's journey to becoming the first woman to earn a medical degree in the United States was fraught with challenges. She was born on February 3, 1821, in Bristol, England. In 1832, her family emigrated to the United States, settling in New York City.

In the 1800s, women were expected to stay within traditional roles, mostly confined to domestic duties. The world of medicine was predominantly male, and this societal barrier made it incredibly difficult for women to pursue a career in the field. Despite these obstacles, Elizabeth was determined to become a physician.

From the start, Elizabeth faced rejection from many medical schools simply because she was a woman. This was a time when educational institutions weren't welcoming to female applicants; women weren't seen as equals to men, especially in rigorous fields like medicine. It seemed almost impossible for a woman to break into this exclusive club.

However, Elizabeth wasn't one to easily give up. She applied to numerous schools, but the norms of the time restricted opportunities for women. The universities' regulations didn't allow women. However, her persistence paid off when Geneva Medical College in New York accepted her application. They didn't really admit her based on her merit, but rather because the male students thought it would be amusing to admit a woman under the assumption that she'd eventually fail. This incident emphasizes how gender bias shaped educational opportunities (Morantz-Sanchez, 1992).

Her acceptance was just the beginning of more trials ahead. Fortunately, amid these setbacks, Elizabeth found support from a community of women who believed in her cause. This network of other women offered her encouragement and mentorship, providing her with the emotional strength needed to forge ahead. Such solidarity was crucial for Elizabeth and many other women of her time who faced discrimination every day.

Once at Geneva Medical College, Elizabeth confronted more discrimination. Her presence in classrooms stirred discomfort among peers and professors who were unaccustomed to a woman's ambition in such venues. Some professors refused to allow her to participate in lectures or practical sessions, limiting opportunities for her to learn. However, Elizabeth chose to persevere, knowing her success would pave the way for others.

Despite these unfavorable conditions, Elizabeth excelled academically. In 1849, she graduated from Geneva Medical College at the top of her class. Her success was nothing short of groundbreaking, offering hope and inspiration to future generations of women aspiring to enter the medical profession. Her graduation wasn't just an individual accomplishment but also a symbol of progress for women's rights, representing a hopeful future where gender wouldn't dictate a person's ability to pursue a career in medicine.

Founding a Medical School for Women

Dr. Elizabeth Blackwell didn't stop after getting her degree; she decided to help other girls achieve their goals. Her belief in women's capability to excel in medical fields was unwavering. Elizabeth stood firm in her conviction that women could match men's achievements in medicine if given equal opportunities. She had succeeded despite all the obstacles she faced, so all girls should have the same chance. Elizabeth was certain that education should be accessible and fair for everyone, regardless of gender.

In 1857, Elizabeth took a monumental step: She established the New York Infirmary for Indigent Women and Children, teaming up with her sister Emily Blackwell and her colleague Dr. Marie Zakrzewska. This institution was revolutionary for its time, providing both healthcare services and educational opportunities exclusively for women. The Infirmary wasn't only a place where female patients could seek medical treatment from women doctors; it was also a critical training ground for female physicians and nurses. This ensured women had full training, equal to men. Elizabeth didn't want future doctors to experience the restrictions she had while studying. This bold move allowed women to gain clinical exposure.

The impact of Blackwell's work extended beyond the establishment of the Infirmary; she was also instrumental in developing a curriculum that emphasized high standards and rigorous education. Blackwell ensured that the courses offered were as challenging and comprehensive as those in any medical school for men. The high standards demonstrated that women could uphold the same, if not higher, academic excellence as their male counterparts, debunking the myth that women couldn't handle the rigors of medical training.

The Women's Medical College of the New York Infirmary opened in 1868. The college was located next to the Infirmary and provided a seamless integration of theoretical learning and practical application. Students could attend classes and immediately apply their knowledge in a clinical setting, preparing them thoroughly for future practice. Emily Blackwell served as the dean, and under her leadership the college gained a reputation for excellence.

Elizabeth Blackwell passed away on May 31, 1910, in Hawthorne, New York, at the age of 89. Her pioneering spirit and relentless advocacy for women's inclusion in medicine illustrate the difference you can make.

Thanks to her efforts, young girls today have more pathways to pursue their dreams in medicine. Elizabeth's legacy continues to inspire, showing us all the importance of pushing boundaries and fighting for equality, ensuring a brighter future for everyone.

The idea of winning a doctor's degree gradually assumed the aspect of a great moral struggle, and the moral fight possessed immense attraction for me.
–Elizabeth Blackwell

Chapter 2:

Virginia Apgar—Advancements in Neonatal Care

Virginia Apgar's journey in neonatal care marked a transformative era in medicine. From an avid learner to a renowned anesthesiologist, Apgar's story showcases her relentless pursuit of knowledge and innovation—a pursuit that eventually led her to introduce the iconic Apgar score. This score allowed doctors to assess critical health indicators in the first minutes of life and forever altered how newborns are assessed right after birth. Apgar's pioneering work changed medical practice and increased life expectancy at birth, a groundbreaking advance in medicine.

Within this chapter, you'll discover the details of how Virginia Apgar found this score and also how she struggled to defeat gender barriers in the field of anesthesiology. She also made significant contributions in this field.

First Woman to Become a Full Professor at Columbia University

Virginia Apgar was born on June 7, 1909, in Westfield, New Jersey. She was the daughter of a successful businessman and a progressive mother, who fostered her interests in education and science from a young age.

Excelling academically, Apgar attended Mount Holyoke College, where she earned her bachelor's degree in 1929.

Virginia was born with an insatiable curiosity and energy. When she grew up, Apgar embarked on a journey that would make her a trailblazer in medicine. After completing medical school at Columbia University's Vagelos College of Physicians and Surgeons in 1933, she became one of the few women in medicine at the time. Her early experiences in medical training motivated her to focus on obstetrics and pediatrics, ultimately leading to her groundbreaking work in neonatal care.

When she was first pursuing her medical career in the 1930s, it was uncommon for women to be seen in leadership positions in medicine. But Apgar was never one to shy away from a challenge. Her first goal was to become a doctor, but she then realized that she wanted to go further. She decided to pivot from surgery to anesthesiology. Women weren't welcomed in surgery rooms; male doctors used to believe women were too sensitive to perform surgery. Virginia didn't listen and instead remained focused on achieving a full professorship in anesthesiology, which was a new field at that time.

This achievement served as an important message to young women everywhere: that they too could aspire to reach the top of their chosen fields, no matter what others told them. Later, Virginia was appointed as the director of the Division of Anesthesia at the Vagelos College of Physicians and Surgeons. She performed there as a clinical instructor and, later, also became the first woman full professor at the institution in 1949 (National Women's Hall of Fame, n.d.).

Throughout her career, Apgar received a great deal of recognition and numerous awards. One such honor was the Gold Medal for Distinguished Achievement in Medicine from Columbia University, reflecting her monumental impact on the field.

Virginia wanted to advocate for maternal and infant health at a national level. She got involved with organizations like the National Foundation (now known as March of Dimes), which allowed her to extend her influence even further. Her role there involved public education and fundraising efforts aimed at reducing birth defects and improving newborn care.

Virginia had a revolutionary idea: She believed that anesthesiologists had to be trained in resuscitation techniques. She was persuaded that this knowledge could save many lives. Once, she said, "Nobody, but nobody, is going to stop breathing on me" (National Women's Hall of Fame, n.d., para. 4). She used to carry a knife and rubber tubes in her bag to be ready in case anyone needed an emergency procedure to allow them to breathe. This simple yet essential first aid kit allowed her to save 16 lives.

Pioneering Anesthesiology in Childbirth

Virginia's journey in medicine began with an incredible impact on anesthesiology, a field that, at the time, lacked specialization for childbirth. Her pioneering work transformed how anesthesia was administered during labor and significantly elevated safety standards for both mothers and newborns. In an era when childbirth complications were common and sometimes fatal, Apgar's innovative techniques brought about a new level of care. Additionally, she added a new perspective on labor: a perspective from another woman, with a deeper understanding of women's pain and concerns.

Apgar developed safer methods for administering anesthesia, particularly focusing on minimizing risks during cesarean deliveries and labor analgesia. Before her interventions, the use of certain drugs often led to dangerous side effects such as respiratory depression (slowed or inadequate breathing) in newborns and complications like maternal aspiration (inhalation of foreign substances, typically gastric contents, into the lungs during pregnancy or childbirth). Virginia studied these effects and worked to improve outcomes, ensuring that anesthesia could be utilized effectively without compromising the health of mothers or babies. This revolution in anesthesia practices meant that more women could choose pain relief during childbirth without additional worry for their safety (Lim et al., 2018).

The Apgar Score

One of Virginia's most renowned contributions to neonatal care was the creation of the Apgar score. While studying and during her years of practice, Virginia learned from keen observation that the first minutes following birth were critical. She realized that swift assessment and intervention could mean the difference between life and death for a newborn.

The Apgar score is a swift assessment given to an infant at one and five minutes following delivery. The score at one minute indicates how well the baby coped with the process of birth. The score at five minutes assesses the baby's condition outside the womb and evaluates their responsiveness in case immediate resuscitation is necessary right after delivery (*Apgar Score*, n.d.).

The Apgar score provided a simple, quick method to evaluate a baby's health immediately after birth, based on five criteria: heart rate, respiration, muscle tone, reflex response, and color. Each element was given a score from zero to two, with a total possible score of ten. This system allowed healthcare professionals to rapidly determine whether a newborn needed immediate medical attention.

Today, the Apgar score may seem intuitive. However, in 1952, when Virginia proposed the score, this procedure wasn't employed by doctors. Thus, the rate of death in newborn children was very high. Virginia knew that the data that could be gathered from the Apgar score would allow doctors to make accurate decisions promptly. It became a universal tool, adopted worldwide, validating the importance of standardized assessments in enhancing newborn survival rates (Ray et al., 2024).

Beyond her technical innovations, Virginia recognized the dire need for comprehensive training among anesthesiologists, particularly in obstetric settings. At the time, many anesthesiologists lacked specific instruction tailored to obstetrics. Apgar fervently advocated for specialized education programs that would equip anesthesiologists with the necessary skills and knowledge to handle the unique challenges of childbirth. She emphasized that well-trained professionals could reduce complications significantly and improve outcomes for mothers and babies.

Besides her contributions to the curricula and practice of anesthesiologists, Virginia claimed that collaboration and teamwork were key to ensuring appropriate healthcare assistance during labor. She encouraged cooperation among obstetricians, pediatricians, and anesthesiologists. This interdisciplinary approach proved crucial in addressing complex medical situations that required integrated expertise. For instance, in high-risk births, having a cohesive team meant that practitioners could anticipate potential complications and respond effectively.

Virginia Apgar's journey provides a powerful example of what's possible when passion meets perseverance. She broke down barriers and set new standards for the early moments of life, changing the world forever. On one occasion, Virginia was asked why she never got married, and she answered...

It's just that I haven't found a man who can cook. –Virginia Apgar

Chapter 3:

Mary Eliza Mahoney—Breaking Down Racial Barriers

Mary Eliza Mahoney's incredible journey as a pioneer in nursing opens a window into the brave strides made by a trailblazer who refused to let obstacles stand in her way. Mary Eliza was an African American citizen who was born into an era fraught with racial discrimination. Nonetheless, she was determined to pursue her dream and serve others.

Let's learn about Mary Eliza's story as the first African American professional nurse and her role in cofounding the National Association of Colored Graduate Nurses (NACGN). Through this organization, she strove to uplift and unite women like her, pushing for equal educational opportunities and fighting against ingrained racial barriers within the healthcare profession. Through Mahoney's life, we're reminded of the power of resilience and its ability to drive progress.

Cofounding the National Association of Colored Graduate Nurses

Mary Eliza Mahoney was born on May 7, 1845, in Boston, Massachusetts. She was the daughter of freed slaves from North Carolina, which influenced her early life and commitment to social justice. Growing up in a region with a growing abolitionist movement, Mahoney developed a strong sense of purpose and determination.

Mary Eliza's commitment to advancing the status of African American nurses was a key part of her groundbreaking career. She recognized that change couldn't be achieved alone but required collective strength and a unified voice. Then, she looked to team up with others, aware that collective efforts are always more effective than individual isolated actions. She was involved in the establishment of the NACGN in 1908, alongside notable figures such as Martha Minerva Franklin and Adah Belle Thoms (Wisconsin Center for Nursing, n.d.). The formation of this organization was vital as it provided a platform for Black nurses to unite and advocate for their rights in a profession dominated by racial inequality.

The NACGN stood at the center of a major fight against discrimination alongside advocacy for deep social reform. One of its primary missions was to fight for equal opportunities in nursing education. At a time when African Americans were often denied access to educational resources, the NACGN championed fair treatment by insisting that Black nurses should receive the same level of training and access to educational materials as their White counterparts. At that time, White and African American people didn't receive equal treatment and had different job and career opportunities. Women could perform as nurses and assist in healthcare centers, but they weren't allowed to obtain a professional credential.

Mary Eliza entered the challenging program to earn a professional nursing license in 1878. She was one of the 42 students who entered the New England Hospital for Women and Children Training School for Nurses in Boston, Massachusetts. Only three students completed the 16-month training program, and Mary Eliza was one of them. After she graduated, she worked as a private duty nurse in Boston (Kays, 2022).

Although Mary Eliza may not have witnessed all the advancements that followed, her groundwork laid the foundation for significant progress in the profession. The perseverance and dedication exemplified by Mary Eliza and other NACGN members echoed through subsequent generations, serving as a powerful reminder of what can be accomplished despite adversity. Their work helped shape policies and attitudes, fostering an environment where excellence isn't limited by race.

Today, organizations, awards, and initiatives honoring minority contributions in nursing reflect Mary Eliza's enduring influence. The sphere of professional development within the nursing community also benefited from Mahoney's efforts. As she and her colleagues pushed for change, they inadvertently established frameworks and networks that facilitated the sharing of knowledge and professional growth among African American nurses. These networks allowed for collaboration and support, significantly improving the professional standing and capabilities of Black nurses during that era.

Networking opportunities, especially those encouraged by associations like the NACGN, proved essential in enabling African American nurses to build relationships, share experiences, and foster mutual advancement.

Advocating for Equality in Nursing Education

Mary Eliza dedicated her life to forging pathways for African American women in the nursing profession. Her efforts were underscored by the myriad obstacles she faced, stemming from systemic barriers within a predominantly White nursing education system (Kays, 2022).

To overcome these hindrances, Mary Eliza focused on public speaking and advocacy. She understood the power of her voice and used it effectively to shine a light on the importance of diversity in healthcare. Public forums became her stage, where she highlighted the significance of having a diverse group of nurses who could offer culturally competent care (Iheduru-Anderson et al., 2022).

Her advocacy contributed to influencing policy changes that would have lasting impacts. Through her efforts, nursing schools gradually began opening their doors to minority students.

The impact of her work is evident today, as her legacy continues to inspire movements dedicated to achieving equity in education (Kays, 2022). Over a century later, we're still fighting against some forms of racial discrimination, but we can celebrate many victories that ensure equal opportunity for us all regardless of our gender and ethnicity. These victories were inspired and started by people like Mary Eliza. Her advocacy and efforts were important for women who wanted to become professional nurses, as well as for patients.

Studies show that patients are more likely to seek preventive medical care when healthcare professionals share their ethnic background. In other words, it was more probable that Black people would seek preventive attention if the nurses were also Black (Kays, 2022). More and better-trained African American nurses meant an improvement in healthcare systems that ensured everybody had equal rights to health.

Mary Eliza Mahoney became the first African American woman to earn a professional nursing credential and, thus, she shattered racial barriers. Her work with the NACGN demonstrated her unwavering commitment to fighting for equal rights in nursing education and practice.

Work more and better the coming year than the previous year.
–Mary Eliza Mahoney

Chapter 4:

Helen Brooke Taussig—Heart Surgery Innovator

Helen Brooke Taussig was particularly concerned about children's health. Her work revolutionized pediatric cardiology during a time when heart surgeries in children were deemed impossible. This narrative dives into her journey, showcasing how her vision led to the development of techniques that would change the face of medical science forever.

You're about to discover the groundbreaking creation of the Blalock–Taussig shunt, a surgical marvel that brought hope to countless families. You'll discover the essential role Taussig played alongside Alfred Blalock and Vivien Thomas in developing this life-saving procedure.

Development and Impact of the Blalock–Taussig Shunt

Helen Brooke Taussig was born on March 24, 1898, in Cambridge, Massachusetts, to a family with a strong academic background. Her father was an architect and her mother was a musician, creating a rich intellectual environment. Taussig faced health challenges early in life, including a serious illness that left her with a lifelong hearing impairment. Despite these obstacles, she pursued her education with determination, earning a degree from Smith College in 1921. Taussig later attended

Johns Hopkins University to study medicine, where she became a pioneer in pediatric cardiology, ultimately founding the field.

In the mid-20th century, Helen emerged as a trailblazer in pediatric cardiology, leaving an indelible mark on medical history. Her critical role in developing the Blalock–Taussig shunt revolutionized the treatment of congenital heart defects in children. Until then, these health issues had been considered beyond the reach of surgical intervention. Before this innovation, many infants with these conditions faced grim prognoses, often unable to survive due to insufficient oxygenated blood circulation.

The Blalock–Taussig shunt was a game-changer. It created a new pathway for blood flow, significantly improving circulation. This new channel connected the subclavian artery to the pulmonary artery, ensuring enough oxygen reached the heart. This innovative approach allowed for increased blood supply to the lungs, enhancing oxygenation and giving babies a fighting chance at life. The procedure offered hope where there had previously been despair.

Helen Taussig collaborated with surgeon Alfred Blalock to bring the shunt to fruition. Their partnership exemplified the immense potential of interdisciplinary teamwork in medicine. Taussig provided the vision and understanding of the cardiac abnormalities affecting these young patients; Blalock on his end brought the procedural expertise needed to turn theory into practice. The duo worked alongside Vivien Thomas, a talented surgical technician whose contributions were vital to the success of the operation. Together, they designed a procedure that saved lives and set a precedent for future collaborations.

The first surgery happened in November 1944 on a 15-month-old baby with a bluish skin tone. No one thought the operation would be successful. It was a very careful and complex procedure that connected the pulmonary artery, which carries blood to the lungs, to another artery that carries oxygen-rich blood. Right after the surgery, it was clear that it had worked: The baby's skin turned pink, and blood flow to the lungs improved (Williamson, 2024).

Through their collaborative efforts, Taussig and her colleagues refined surgical techniques that would go on to impact countless families worldwide. The Blalock–Taussig shunt became a cornerstone of pediatric cardiac surgery, laying down principles and standards that are still referenced in modern times.

It also laid the groundwork for future advancements in pediatric heart surgery. The technique demonstrated that complex heart conditions in children could be managed surgically, inspiring generations of medical professionals to push the boundaries of what was thought possible.

Even decades after its inception, the Blalock–Taussig shunt remains a crucial tool in treating certain congenital heart defects, a testament to its lasting influence.

Research on Thalidomide and Advocacy for Child Health

Helen also carried out research into the effects of thalidomide. Thalidomide was initially developed in Germany during the late 1950s and early 1960s as a treatment for morning sickness in pregnant women, and was used as a sedative to treat nausea. It was widely considered safe. However, it later became linked to serious birth defects, sparking a crisis that demanded immediate attention. Children were born with malformations of their hands and fingers, damage to their eyes and ears, and even problems with their brains and bones (The Thalidomide Trust, n.d.).

Helen recognized an alarming pattern through her rigorous research. She identified a direct connection between thalidomide usage and congenital heart defects in newborns. This pivotal discovery led to widespread discussions about drug safety during pregnancy, drawing attention to the potential hazards pharmaceuticals could pose to unborn children. Helen's work raised awareness among medical professionals and the public, highlighting the need for the more stringent evaluation of drugs intended for pregnant women (Williamson, 2024).

After her discovery, Helen continued advocating for stricter regulations on medications given to expectant mothers. She shared her findings with authorities like the U.S. Food and Drug Administration (FDA) and helped foster a movement toward ethical considerations in healthcare. Her efforts were instrumental in preventing the widespread distribution of thalidomide in the United States, saving countless lives from being affected by the drug's devastating consequences (Elliott, 2017).

Upon her return to the United States in 1962, Taussig presented her research and provided testimony to the American College of Physicians and Congress, highlighting the dangers associated with thalidomide. Her compelling evidence and persuasive arguments led to the drug's prohibition in the US. Furthermore, her work prompted President Kennedy and the FDA to implement enhanced drug testing protocols aimed at understanding the impact of medications on birth defects (Elliott, 2017). Alongside colleagues like Dr. Frances Oldham Kelsey (see Chapter 15), Taussig's relentless pursuit of ethical accountability reshaped how pharmaceutical companies approach drug testing and approval processes, particularly concerning pregnant women.

Helen actively engaged in lecturing and travel to disseminate her knowledge. Her lectures put the issue of drug safety under the spotlight, educating both medical communities and the public about the importance of protecting vulnerable populations such as pregnant women and newborn babies.

She officially stepped down from her role at Johns Hopkins in 1963, yet she remained dedicated to her research and passionately championed the field of pediatric cardiology. In 1964, President Lyndon Johnson awarded her the Presidential Medal of Freedom for her significant contributions to treating and preventing heart disease in children. In 1965, she became both the first woman and the first pediatric cardiologist to lead the American Heart Association. Additionally, in 1976 she was inducted into the National Academy of Arts and Sciences.

Helen Brooke Taussig's groundbreaking development of the Blalock–Taussig shunt transformed pediatric heart surgery and inspired future medical advances. Yet her contributions didn't stop there. Her dedication to child health extended into advocacy, as seen in her critical research on thalidomide. By uncovering thalidomide's harmful effects, she highlighted the importance of drug safety for pregnant women, protecting countless families from potential tragedies.

Learn to listen with your fingers. –Helen Brooke Taussig

Chapter 5:

Florence Nightingale—

Establishing Modern Nursing

Florence Nightingale's work in modern nursing began in 1853, during the Crimean War. Working in military hospitals, she faced dire sanitary conditions that endangered soldiers' lives. Amid these challenges, Florence implemented groundbreaking changes in healthcare procedures, emphasizing the importance of cleanliness and hygiene. She brought attention to the critical link between sanitary conditions and patient survival.

Her observations and findings resulted in sweeping reforms within the British Army and beyond, highlighting her influence on healthcare policies worldwide.

Revolutionizing Hospital Sanitation Practices

Florence Nightingale was born on May 12, 1820, in Florence, Italy, to affluent British parents. Raised in a privileged environment, she received a strong education that allowed her to showcase her intelligence from a young age. Nightingale was deeply influenced by her family's emphasis on social responsibility and philanthropy. Despite societal expectations for women of her class to marry and lead a domestic life, she felt a calling to nursing.

During the Crimean War, Florence Nightingale arrived at the military hospital in Scutari, Turkey, to find appalling sanitary conditions. The soldiers there were not only battling injuries from the war but also suffering due to inadequate hygiene practices. The lack of clean linen, proper drainage, and basic necessities like soap and towels contributed to a grim environment where diseases such as typhus, cholera, and dysentery claimed more lives than the actual combat wounds (Fee & Garofalo, 2010). This harrowing experience fueled Florence's determination to advocate for better hygiene and sanitation standards.

In the mid-19th century, the scientific method was still under development. There were many things that were still unknown. Despite this, Florence was able to recognize the power of data and became a pioneer in using statistical evidence, recording data to highlight the critical link between sanitary conditions and mortality rates. She meticulously collected data during her time at Scutari, revealing that a large number of deaths would have been preventable if proper sanitation measures had been implemented. Her famous "coxcomb" diagrams visually demonstrated how improvements in cleanliness dramatically decreased death rates. This innovative use of statistics strengthened her arguments; moreover, it laid the foundation for new approaches in medicine based on facts and evidence (Aravind & Chung, 2010).

These findings were used to make significant changes to the management of medical procedures within the British Army. Florence was one of the founders of the Royal Commission on the Health of the Army, which conducted thorough investigations into the state of military hospitals. Through her detailed reports and recommendations, the Commission implemented extensive reforms, including improved ventilation systems, cleaner facilities, and better nutrition for patients. These reforms had a profound impact. The number of deaths reduced and recovery processes improved as medical teams implemented new standards for military healthcare practices.

The changes inspired by Nightingale's work extended far beyond the immediate context of military hospitals. Her principles of cleanliness, organization, and compassionate care also reached civilian healthcare systems all over the world. By demonstrating how thoughtful hygienic practices could save lives, she influenced global health policies. Her approach emphasized prevention over treatment, highlighting that a healthy environment was key to warding off disease.

It's interesting to notice that, 170 years later, hygienic practices continue to be critical to stopping infection and enhancing recovery treatments. During the Covid-19 pandemic, extreme hygienic practices were the cornerstone to dealing with this potentially deadly unknown virus.

The Nightingale Training School for Nurses

Florence Nightingale, recognized as the pioneer of modern nursing, is strongly linked to St Thomas' Hospital in London, UK. In 1859, she authored a significant work titled *Notes on Nursing*, which addressed the care of the ill. Her goal was to elevate nursing into a respectable profession for women, grounded in a rigorous training approach centered on commitment and discipline.

Supported by St Thomas' Court of Governors and an impressive fund of nearly £50,000, the Nightingale Training School for Nurses—the world's first institution of its kind—began operations at St Thomas' in 1860. Florence appointed Mrs. Sarah Wardroper, who had served as matron since 1854, as the School's inaugural superintendent. All nursing students and certified Nightingale nurses resided in the Nightingale Home, wore uniforms, and were required to follow a stringent ethical code (Guy's and St Thomas' NHS Foundation Trust, n.d.).

Florence's greatest achievement was developing a structured curriculum that combined practical skills with theoretical knowledge. She believed that nurses should be well-rounded professionals capable of providing exceptional patient care, which meant they needed both hands-on experience and a strong educational foundation.

The creation of this comprehensive training program was groundbreaking at the time. Nursing students learned about anatomy, hygiene, disease prevention, and the best practices for patient care. This balanced approach equipped them with the necessary tools to save lives and improve community health standards.

In addition to these educational innovations, Nightingale championed the empowerment of women through nursing. At a time when career paths for women were extremely limited, she opened doors that had previously been closed to them. Her School offered women the opportunity to learn and work as professional nurses, breaking into a field largely dominated by men. Her work showed that women could excel in challenging and demanding professions, encouraging others to strive for similar opportunities.

Furthermore, Florence introduced the Nightingale Pledge, which embodies ethical practice and professionalism in nursing. It's a solemn promise that serves as a reminder of the responsibilities nurses have toward their patients. It emphasizes the importance of compassion, confidentiality, accountability, and lifelong learning. By taking the pledge, nurses committed themselves not only to the technical aspects of their jobs but also to adhering to high moral and ethical standards. The Nightingale Pledge affirms the noble ideals that guide nurses in their endeavors.

Florence Nightingale's impact on healthcare and nursing improved hospital sanitation during the Crimean War. Eventually, this transformed how hospitals operate, saving countless lives by emphasizing cleanliness and hygiene. Her introduction of data-driven approaches laid the groundwork for modern healthcare practices and inspired changes that rippled through medical institutions worldwide.

A hundred struggle and drown in the breakers. One discovers the new world. Rather, ten times, die in the surf heralding the way to a new world, than stand idly on the shore. –Florence Nightingale

Chapter 6:

Mary Breckinridge—Healthcare in Appalachia

Mary Breckinridge had a vision that helped change healthcare in remote areas of the US, especially Appalachia. Mary began by exploring different ways to help mothers and babies stay healthy, inspired by her experiences overseas. She realized that combining Native American traditions with modern medicine could make a big difference when medical care was out of reach. Mary worked tirelessly to bring high-quality care to rural communities.

Below, you'll learn about the bold steps Mary took to introduce nurse-midwifery in the United States. By establishing training programs for nurse-midwives, she addressed the lack of trained healthcare professionals in rural areas. You'll also discover this visionary leader who transformed public health in the US and inspired similar efforts worldwide.

Introduction of Nurse-Midwifery to the US

Mary Breckinridge was born on February 17, 1881, in Memphis, Tennessee, into a prominent Southern family. She faced personal tragedy early in life, including the deaths of her mother and two children, which deeply impacted her perspectives on healthcare. Educated at private schools and later at the University of Tennessee, Breckinridge sought a more meaningful path than just being a housewife.

Mary had a curious spirit and wanted to see the world. She embarked on a journey to Europe and spent some time there exploring midwifery techniques. When she came back to the United States, she thought that similar techniques would be beneficial for communities settled in rural areas. People living there didn't have access to healthcare. Native American communities, however, had their own traditional midwifery. Mary understood that both medical practices could be blended to address critical health needs in underserved areas. By integrating the best of both worlds, Mary developed a unique approach that would become the cornerstone of her work in Appalachia.

Mary started working to improve healthcare access in rural communities in the US. The lack of trained healthcare professionals posed a significant challenge in these regions. Then, she established rigorous training programs for nurse-midwives. These programs were pioneering, addressing the workforce shortages typical of rural areas. Mary's initiative created a new generation of nurse-midwives so the most isolated individuals could access professional medical attention.

These nurse-midwives weren't merely healthcare providers; they became integral members of their communities. They engaged in the cultural nuances and traditions of the people they served. Mary believed that what these communities needed was more than just medical attention; they needed people who understood and were respectful of their culture, because that would enable them to trust. You won't heal if you can't trust your medical care provider. By respecting local customs, these nurse-midwives established strong bonds with families, breaking down barriers that often hindered access to healthcare.

The Breckinridge model had a broader impact. It was initially targeted at rural communities, but was later implemented in modern midwifery practices. Her strategies and methodologies continue to influence approaches to maternity care and community health today.

Mary introduced a new approach to healthcare. She believed that besides treating patients, healthcare should support holistic well-being. Her work highlighted the importance of continuity in care, a principle that remains relevant today. Also, she showcased how to take healthcare to rural areas and reduce logistical barriers so everybody can get accurate medical assistance.

Mary's efforts contributed to elevating the role of nurse-midwives and giving more social value to the profession. Nurse-midwives play a key role in healthcare and are the ones who stand closest to patients during treatment and recovery. By demonstrating the value of systematic training and culturally sensitive practices, she set a precedent for other healthcare fields, leading to a re-evaluation of how healthcare can be delivered effectively in various contexts.

Improving Maternal and Infant Health Outcomes

In 1925, Mary founded the Frontier Nursing Service (FNS) to work with communities in Appalachia. She revolutionized rural healthcare, with a focus on reducing maternal and infant mortality rates. Her efforts were very important because her interventions effectively lowered the number of children's and mothers' deaths at birth.

Mary's approach was innovative for its time. Native American communities lived close to the frontiers with few roads, limited means of communication, and a less developed medical assistance system. Mary ensured that women in these communities received both prenatal and postnatal care directly at their homes. This personalized attention provided timely medical intervention and increased access to essential healthcare services.

The convenience and comfort of receiving care at home meant that more women participated in the program. This allowed them to remain healthier during pregnancy and reach the moment of labor in better health, also ensuring the baby's health. This model of care highlighted how crucial it is to make healthcare accessible, especially in remote areas where traditional medical facilities are scarce or inaccessible. By bringing healthcare to the doorsteps of those who needed it most, Mary made an indelible mark on public health practices.

An essential facet of Mary's strategy was community health education, another innovative idea for the time. The FNS program included teaching local communities about important aspects of maternal health, nutrition, and child care. Education empowers individuals to take charge of their own health and well-being. Understanding proper nutrition and child-rearing practices helped families make informed decisions, contributing to a healthier lifestyle. With simple techniques and accessible language, Mary made sure that the information was understandable to everyone, thus ensuring inclusivity in health education.

Mary was a pioneer in working collaboratively with local leaders and engaging with grassroots movements. These partnerships were instrumental in building trust between the FNS and the communities it served. Local leaders acted as bridges, conveying the needs and concerns of the population to the nurses and midwives, while also advocating for the program and its benefits. Through these collaborations, the FNS was able to tailor its initiatives to better meet the specific needs of each community. This grassroots approach demonstrated how involving community members in health initiatives could enable success.

Mary's vision led to reduced maternal and infant mortality rates, showing how personalized care could transform lives. Her work highlighted the importance of adapting healthcare systems to meet local needs.

Work for children should begin before they are born... These are the formative years, whether for their bodies, their minds or their loving hearts. –Mary Breckinridge

Chapter 7:

Mary Woodard Lasker—Impact on Cancer Research Pioneer

Mary Woodard Lasker played a significant role in changing how we understand and treat cancer today. Her forward-thinking ideas led her to raise funds to improve biological therapies. With her contributions, she helped shift the focus from traditional methods like surgery and radiation to more innovative treatments that harness the body's natural defenses. Her contributions led to the exploration of the complex biology of how cancer grows and spreads, paving the way for breakthroughs with a lasting impact.

In this chapter, you'll learn about how Mary fostered collaboration to achieve remarkable advancements in cancer research. You'll explore how she set up clinical trials to turn scientific discoveries into real-life changes that could benefit patients.

Founding a Cancer Research Institute

Mary was devoted to finding new alternatives to treat cancer. Her work was characterized by an unwavering commitment to support research on the biological factors that contribute to cancer development and progression. Examining how these biological factors influence cancer opened new pathways for treatment. Mary's efforts focused on teams working to understand the intricate interactions within the body. This helped doctors identify potential targets for innovative therapies. These groundbreaking discoveries enabled other researchers to explore cancer's complexities in depth.

One of Lasker's most significant contributions was engaging in research programs that challenged conventional methods of treating diseases. When she started working, treatments were often limited to surgery and radiation. Instead, Mary supported researchers who explored the potential of harnessing the body's natural defenses. This was a radical idea then, as it suggested that the immune system could be used to combat cancer.

Before this new approach, the immune system was long viewed as a protective shield against infections but wasn't considered as a resource for disease treatment. Then, Mary's institute promoted the concept of immunotherapy, shifting the paradigm toward more personalized and targeted approaches.

Lasker's foundation enabled pioneering work in clinical trials, marking another milestone in cancer research. She recognized the importance of translating scientific discoveries into practical applications that could directly benefit patients. To this end, researchers initiated and conducted early-stage clinical trials, rigorously testing the safety and efficacy of new therapies. These trials provided valuable insights and laid the foundation for developing more effective treatments. Her efforts reduced the gap between laboratory research and real-world application to ensure that scientific advancements reached those who needed them most (Levy, 2023).

Through these pioneering initiatives, Mary left a profound legacy in biological research. Her vision to support the search for understanding biological factors reshaped treatment strategies and encouraged continuous exploration beyond traditional boundaries. Today's emerging technologies and scientific advancements continue to build upon her foundation.

Founding a Cancer Research Institute

In 1942, Mary and her husband Albert Lasker, a successful advertising pioneer, started the Lasker Foundation to advance medical research. Lasker also played a key role in transforming the American Cancer Society into a powerful organization that could effectively advocate for more funding for cancer research from Congress.

She was among the first to champion cancer chemotherapy, encouraging scientists to move their discoveries into drug production faster. She also pushed for the creation of the National Heart Institute (NHI), which is now known as the National Heart, Lung, and Blood Institute, and the National Institute of Mental Health. Lasker made sure that regular people were included on NHI scientific advisory boards, a position she often took on herself. Congressional leaders trusted her expert witnesses when it came time to argue for significant increases in the NHI budget every year.

One of Mary's most significant achievements was the establishment of an institute dedicated to research. This effort went beyond scientific inquiry: She wanted to ensure that her ideas would be deepened and bring more innovations to the field.

Mary believed that the most important thing was to create a nourishing environment for researchers to work collaboratively. She made sure to instill her values in her teams. Nonetheless, it was also critical to build facilities and acquire high-tech equipment to ease the research. Thus, she had to sort out the obstacle of raising funds. She skillfully navigated the complexities of obtaining funds from various sources, ensuring that the Lasker Foundation could support novel projects and research initiatives. The funding she secured financed equipment and facilities and allowed for an influx of talented scientists. They were driven by the desire to contribute to the field but also to be members of Mary's team.

Moreover, Mary was able to secure permanent funding. Research, particularly in fields as intricate as cancer biology, requires sustained investment. Such financial support enables teams to explore, experiment, and eventually discover groundbreaking treatments (Liao et al., 2024).

Beyond funding and infrastructure, fostering the next generation of scientists was another pillar of Lasker's approach. She opened training programs and mentorship opportunities. Her foundation became a fertile ground for aspiring researchers, who could learn from established experts and develop their skills in a supportive environment.

These training and educational opportunities were instrumental in providing young scientists with the hands-on experience they needed. At the foundation, interns and trainees could engage in real-world research, contributing to meaningful projects while learning the intricacies of scientific investigation.

In 1945, Albert and Mary Lasker launched the Lasker Awards to highlight groundbreaking biological research and medical innovations that enhance human well-being. This initiative also emphasizes the crucial role of public backing for scientific endeavors. This foundation is considered the top honor in biomedical research in the US. Amazingly, over 70 recipients of this prize have gone on to win Nobel Prizes.

Mary developed revolutionary biological therapies that harnessed the natural defenses of the human body and paved the way for cancer treatments that are still used today. Her ideas brought a breeze of hope for patients and families struggling with this difficult disease and opened the door to other approaches to treatment.

Nobody would have me in their laboratory for five minutes. I couldn't cut up a frog, and I certainly couldn't perform surgery. I'm better at making it possible for other people. –Mary Woodard Lasker

Chapter 8:

Tu Youyou—Saving Lives With Artemisinin

Tu Youyou's pioneering discovery of artemisinin marked a turning point in the treatment of malaria, showcasing the intersection of traditional knowledge and modern scientific inquiry. Her work transformed medical practices and highlighted the determined pursuit of innovation.

Below, you'll read about the significance of Tu Youyou's Nobel Prize win and its global recognition as a pivotal moment in medical history. Her discoveries had a profound impact on public health worldwide, particularly in reducing malaria-related mortality rates. Moreover, you'll learn about Tu's leadership during the turbulent Cultural Revolution, where she guided a team through adversity to scientific triumph.

Nobel Prize in Physiology or Medicine

Malaria is a life-threatening disease caused by parasites transmitted through the bites of infected female *Anopheles* mosquitoes. It leads to symptoms such as fever, chills, and flu-like illness and can result in severe complications or death if not treated promptly.

In the 1960s, malaria was a significant public health challenge in China, especially in rural areas. The disease caused substantial morbidity and mortality, affecting millions of people. The government launched extensive campaigns to control malaria, including efforts to drain swamps, improve sanitation, and distribute insecticide-treated bed nets. By the end of the decade, these measures had led to a marked decline in malaria cases, showcasing the effectiveness of public health interventions in combating the disease.

In 2015, Tu Youyou became the first Chinese scientist from the mainland to receive the Nobel Prize, which she was awarded in Physiology or Medicine. This was a remarkable achievement that celebrated her groundbreaking work in discovering artemisinin, a revolutionary drug that transformed how the world treats malaria. The Nobel Prize is one of the highest honors in the global scientific community, given only to those whose contributions significantly push the boundaries of knowledge and improve human life (Liu & Liu, 2016).

Youyou's discovery of artemisinin has saved millions of lives across the globe. Malaria is rampant in many regions of the world, including many developing countries, even at present. Before her breakthrough, malaria claimed the lives of hundreds of thousands each year. However, with artemisinin-based therapies, mortality rates have dropped dramatically (Liu & Liu, 2016).

Artemisinin is a plant that grows in China and has been used for medicinal purposes for centuries. The use of this plant wasn't part of Western medicine but belonged to the rich heritage of traditional Chinese medicine. Tu sought a way to combine the best of both worlds, devoting herself to using this plant with well-known properties to manufacture medicine in the laboratory. When she and her team isolated artemisinin from sweet wormwood, they discovered an effective weapon against malaria that outperformed existing treatments in both speed and effectiveness (*Tu Youyou*, n.d.). The direct impact of this discovery is evident in improved health outcomes and countless lives saved worldwide.

Tu Youyou's discovery and her popularity have sparked discussions about the importance of investing in scientific research and improving the protection of intellectual property rights, particularly in her homeland, China. These factors are important to encourage more researchers to work on innovation and ensure that the fruits of their scientific labor are recognized and rewarded. China continues to reform its scientific research system (Liu & Liu, 2016).

Leading a Team During the Cultural Revolution

Tu Youyou wasn't only a medical researcher busy in her lab. When the Cultural Revolution broke out in China, she became the leader of a research team. While the country was dragged into a long and violent period of political instability, she continued to attend to people's health.

The Cultural Revolution started in 1966 and was a period of significant cultural and political turmoil in China. Mao Zedong, the chairman of the Communist Party, sought to reinforce communist ideologies and wanted to destroy all elements perceived as bourgeois or counter-revolutionary. The revolution was against capitalism. But Zedong didn't only want to keep power; he wanted everything in society to be aligned with the Communist Party's ideas.

Among the institutions affected by Zedong's orders were universities and research centers; academic and scientific endeavors were seriously hampered. Many intellectuals and scientists found their work interrupted or redirected under government mandates. Framed by this challenging context, Tu Youyou was able to spearhead efforts in traditional Chinese medicine research. Her task was to discover an antimalarial treatment.

Youyou didn't work alone. Her team worked hard on the process of discovering how to use artemisinin to treat malaria. The initial experiments were promising, but some inconsistent results challenged their findings. Instead of giving up, Youyou motivated her team to continue through methodical approaches. They refined their extraction methods, going back to ancient texts and modernizing their interpretations with rigorous testing.

As a female leader in a predominantly male domain, particularly within the constraints of her era, Tu Youyou's role transcended mere scientific innovation. Her position was emblematic of changing tides in gender recognition within science, especially in a strongly conservative society such as China during the Cultural Revolution.

Tu Youyou's work on artemisinin demonstrated groundbreaking scientific achievement and highlighted the power of combining traditional knowledge with modern science. This incredible blend was key for making an impact on healthcare worldwide.

When you are entrusted with an assignment, you do your best. –Tu Youyou

Chapter 9:

Patricia Bath—Visionary in Ophthalmology

Transforming the field of ophthalmology, Patricia Bath emerged as a visionary in medical history. Her groundbreaking work resulted in the development of devices for cataract surgery that revolutionized eye care globally.

This chapter explores the inspiring journey of Dr. Bath and her remarkable achievements. As an African American woman striving for recognition in a field dominated by race and gender barriers, her professional career in medicine was filled with struggles that she overcame.

First African American Woman to Receive a Medical Patent

Imagine living in a time when securing a patent, especially in the medical field, was akin to climbing a steep mountain. In the early 1980s, the landscape of medical patents was often riddled with societal obstacles, making it difficult for many inventors to gain recognition for their innovations. These challenges were even more pronounced for women and, specifically, African American women like Patricia Bath.

Throughout the history of medical patents, women have faced many barriers. For an African American woman, these challenges were multiplied, considering the racial prejudices that existed. The system was unwelcoming, and there were very few role models to follow. Yet Patricia didn't allow these hurdles to deter her ambition.

After struggling against all types of obstacles, Patricia obtained the patent for her invention, the Laserphaco Probe. The Laserphaco Probe is a medical device used in ophthalmic surgery, specifically for the treatment of cataracts.

Cataracts are a common eye condition where the clear lens of the eye becomes cloudy or blurry, making it hard to see. Imagine looking through a foggy window—that's what it can feel like for someone with cataracts. Cataracts often develop slowly as people get older, but they can also be caused by factors like genetics, injury, or certain medications. The good news is that cataracts can be treated with surgery, where the cloudy lens is removed and replaced with a clear artificial lens, helping people see clearly again.

Patricia's invention utilized laser technology to break up and remove cloudy lens material from the eye, allowing for the insertion of an artificial lens. The Laserphaco Probe was designed to perform this procedure with precision and minimal damage to the surrounding tissues, promoting quicker recovery times for patients. Its use represented an advancement in cataract surgery, offering an alternative to traditional techniques that employed ultrasound.

Her invention revolutionized cataract surgery, employing a minimally invasive technique that leveraged laser technology to restore vision. This invention improved the quality of life for many people across the globe. Patricia also went further by advocating for the adoption and implementation of her techniques worldwide. Her efforts ensured that millions of patients benefited from modern cataract treatment procedures.

Cofounding the American Institute for the Prevention of Blindness

Patricia's dedication to public health and preventive medicine is evident in her remarkable achievements and the influential roles she played throughout her career. One of her most significant contributions was cofounding the American Institute for the Prevention of Blindness (AiPB) in 1977. This organization was established with a clear mission: to promote eye health awareness through education and to assert that eyesight is a basic human right. The AiPB was committed to ensuring that eye care would become an integral part of basic healthcare services available to everyone, regardless of their economic status.

Since her days as a student, Patricia had noticed that there were deep disparities in eye care services among different populations. As a health professional, she knew the importance of access to healthcare services. During her early research years at Columbia University, she noticed significantly higher rates of blindness and visual impairment among patients at Harlem Hospital compared to those at the Columbia Eye Clinic. This discovery moved her to address these inequalities by improving access to eye care services for underserved populations.

A key strategy employed by Patricia and the AiPB involved educational outreach programs designed to improve public knowledge about eye health. These programs aimed to provide practical solutions that empowered individuals to take charge of their eye health. By spreading awareness, the AiPB ensured that communities were informed about preventive measures, the symptoms of potential eye diseases, and the importance of regular checkups. Such initiatives were especially crucial in educating people on how to protect their vision and prevent avoidable blindness.

These outreach programs often included the training of ophthalmic assistants who could offer basic eye care services and education in various communities. Thus, Patricia's team equipped local healthcare providers with the necessary knowledge and skills. In this way, they were able to educate members of the community and provide them with immediate basic assistance when advanced medical facilities were lacking.

The impact of Bath's advocacy extends far beyond her lifetime. The principles she championed—education, accessibility, prevention—remain important today, being at the core of integral medicine. The AiPB continues to support global initiatives such as providing protective anti-infection eye drops to newborns, administering vitamin A supplements to malnourished children, and vaccinating against diseases like measles, which can lead to blindness. These programs are testaments to her enduring legacy and reinforce the idea that preventive measures are crucial in combating health issues.

Patricia Bath's invention of the Laserphaco Probe reshaped cataract surgery. By cofounding the AiPB, she worked tirelessly to make eye care accessible to everyone. Her advocacy work ensured that awareness and preventive measures reached underserved communities, emphasizing that healthcare is a right, not a privilege.

Believe in the power of truth. Do not allow your mind to be imprisoned by majority thinking. Remember that the limits of science are not the limits of imagination. |
–Patricia Bath

Chapter 10:

Sister Elizabeth Kenny—Polio Treatment Trailblazer

Sister Elizabeth Kenny's revolutionary approach to polio treatment redefined what medical innovation could achieve during the early 20th century. Entering a field governed by entrenched practices wasn't easy, yet Sister Kenny boldly stepped into this world. The prevailing techniques at the time revolved around immobilizing the affected limbs, using braces and splints to prevent movement under the belief that it would aid healing.

However, Sister Elizabeth saw the flaws in these methods and dared to challenge them with her pioneering ideas. Her work demonstrated that there are always new ways to tackle old problems if you have the courage to think differently. By focusing on muscle strength instead of inactivity, she opened up possibilities for recovery that had previously been thought unattainable.

Her methods provided hope to many who were resigned to a future limited by disability—despite the significant opposition she faced from the established medical community, who often viewed her as a rebel.

Challenging Established Medical Practices

Sister Elizabeth Kenny entered the world of medicine at a time when traditional approaches to treating polio were firmly entrenched. Her entry into this field was nothing short of audacious.

Polio, short for poliomyelitis, is a viral disease that can affect the nervous system and lead to paralysis. It spreads mainly through contaminated food and water. In the early 20th century, polio outbreaks were common, especially during the summer months, causing fear and concern for families. Many young people were affected, and some were left with lifelong disabilities. The disease could also be fatal in severe cases.

In the early 20th century, polio became a significant public health concern, especially during the summer months when outbreaks occurred. The virus primarily affected children and could lead to paralysis or even death. High-profile cases, including that of U.S. President Franklin D. Roosevelt, heightened public awareness and fear of the disease. Before the development of vaccines, polio epidemics led to widespread panic, prompting communities to implement quarantines and other measures to control the spread. The disease peaked in the United States during the 1940s and 1950s, with thousands of cases reported annually

The introduction of the polio vaccine had to wait until the 1950s, when it significantly reduced the number of polio cases; today, polio has been almost completely eradicated in many parts of the world due to vaccination efforts. However, in the early 20th century, polio treatment followed a rigid methodology that primarily relied on immobilization techniques.

These methods often involved placing patients in splints or braces to prevent movement and further damage, which was believed necessary for healing. Sister Kenny faced these outdated practices head-on with bravery and determination, challenging the status quo and fighting for innovative treatments.

Her methodology was centered on an unconventional idea at the time: focusing on muscle strength rather than immobilization. Instead of using devices to restrict movement, she advocated for gentle exercise and muscle stimulation. This approach aimed to maintain muscle tone and promote blood flow, which she believed would aid recovery and prevent permanent disability. Her method was particularly significant because it directly influenced patient outcomes, providing hope for many who had previously been resigned to a limited future. By choosing to stimulate the muscles actively, Sister Kenny offered patients a chance at recovery and a return to normal life.

The incorporation of hot packs and targeted exercises in her treatments was revolutionary. It provided patients with immediate relief and significantly improved their long-term prospects (*10 Women Who've Transformed Healthcare in Australia*, n.d.). Her focus on keeping patients engaged and active, both physically and mentally, was a stark contrast to the passive care they were used to receiving. These methods resulted in better physical health and boosted patients' morale, offering them a more optimistic outlook on their condition. Bear in mind that at this time, science hadn't yet explained the close connection between mental and physical health. Sister Kenny was a visionary.

Despite her impactful work, she encountered significant backlash from the medical establishment. Many physicians and scientists dismissed her theories, especially those suggesting polio was not a strictly neurological disease (Rogers, 2014). This skepticism was fueled by deeply rooted beliefs in traditional practices, and many saw her as a rule-breaker more than a trailblazer. However, Sister Kenny remained steadfast in her convictions. Her resilience in facing criticism and opposition highlighted her determination and commitment to improving patient care.

The integration of Sister Kenny's practices into medical training marked a turning point, signifying her far-reaching influence on the field of medicine. Over time, healthcare professionals began adopting her techniques, recognizing the benefits they provided to patients. Her methodologies became foundational elements in rehabilitation training programs, reshaping how polio and similar conditions were approached. Her legacy continued to shape medical practice.

Global Expansion and Advocacy

Sister Elizabeth Kenny decided to open clinics in various parts of the world. She aimed to provide accessible healthcare to polio patients and train other practitioners in her innovative techniques. Through these clinics, she provided direct care to countless individuals and also equipped many other medical professionals with the skills necessary to continue her work, multiplying her impact across continents.

Sister Kenny progressively gained global recognition for her methods. Despite facing initial skepticism from the medical community, especially due to her lack of formal medical training, her persistence and proven results gradually won her widespread acclaim. By securing support from influential organizations and hospitals, including the Minnesota Health Department, she was able to establish her clinics in the United States (Cartwright, 2012). Her methods were also adopted by numerous clinics worldwide.

Sister Elizabeth Kenny's groundbreaking methods in polio treatment brought a new wave of hope to countless patients who had been trapped by outdated medical practices. She managed to transform skepticism into acceptance and respect. Her clinics created a legacy that transcends cultural borders, continuing to inspire new generations of doctors and health professionals.

> *At first, I was called a quack, a charlatan, and worse, year after year, in Australia, England and the United States, by men who simply refused to believe that a nurse from "the bush" could devise a treatment which succeeded where they had failed.* –Sister Elizabeth Kenny

Chapter 11:

Nancy Wexler—Mapping Genetic Disease

This chapter explores Nancy Wexler's pioneering role in unraveling the complexities of Huntington's disease, a hereditary condition that has long puzzled scientists and devastated families worldwide. Nancy's unique blend of scientific rigor and humanity has shed light on the genetic mechanisms behind this disorder and laid the groundwork for discussions on ethical conduct in genetic research.

Nancy contributed to genetic research, particularly through her work with a Venezuelan community near Lake Maracaibo. From traversing challenging terrains to navigating political and social landscapes, each step of her journey highlights her dedication and ingenuity.

The Venezuelan Study of Huntington's Disease

Nancy's journey into the realm of genetic research began with an incredible mission in Venezuela. She dedicated much of her life to studying Huntington's disease, a genetic disorder that causes the progressive breakdown of nerve cells in the brain. It affects movement, cognition, and mood, leading to symptoms such as involuntary jerking or writhing movements (chorea), difficulty with coordination, and cognitive decline. The disease is caused by a mutation in the *HTT* gene, which leads to the production of a toxic protein that damages brain cells.

Symptoms usually appear in mid-adulthood, but they can vary widely in onset and severity.

She was particularly interested in how the disease impacted a small community near Lake Maracaibo, Venezuela, in South America. This area was home to one of the largest clusters of Huntington's disease patients globally. The genetic uniqueness of this community offered scientists a rare opportunity to map the disease and its inheritance patterns with remarkable clarity (Hernandez et al., 2024). The work done here wasn't just about collecting data; it was about understanding the lives affected by this hereditary condition and finding ways to improve them.

Wexler's innovative approach to data collection played a crucial role in the success of this project. Unlike traditional methods, her techniques respected and prioritized the rights and dignity of the participants. Her team employed participatory research practices, which are approaches that actively involve community members or stakeholders in the research process. Instead of researchers just collecting data and making decisions on their own, they collaborate with the people who are affected by the issues being studied. This way, Nancy's team ensured that those involved were informed and consented at every stage.

This approach upheld high ethical standards and fostered trust between the researchers and the community, leading to more accurate and meaningful data. Effective data collection goes beyond gathering information to involve building relationships and respecting participants' humanity, particularly when talking about sensitive topics such as health (International Parkinson and Movement Disorder Society, 2023).

Nancy's team faced several difficulties in accessing remote areas and navigating political tensions. The regions around Lake Maracaibo were often isolated, lacking basic infrastructure such as roads, electricity, and healthcare facilities. Getting there meant traversing long distances on rough terrain, which required careful planning and immense perseverance. Despite these obstacles, Nancy never wavered. She maneuvered through complex social landscapes, respecting local customs and working alongside Venezuelan scientists who provided invaluable insights and support.

This research significantly advanced our understanding of Huntington's disease and paved the way for developing genetic testing and counseling practices. By identifying the genetic markers associated with Huntington's, Nancy contributed to breakthroughs that allowed families to make informed decisions about their health and future (Hernandez et al., 2024).

Advocating for Genetic Testing Guidelines

One of Nancy's most significant accomplishments is the development of comprehensive guidelines that ensure ethical treatment in genetic testing. This involves a keen focus on informed consent and transparency as a means to safeguard individuals undergoing genetic testing. Informed consent is all about making sure people understand what they're signing up for when they agree to genetic tests. This can involve explaining the risks, benefits, and potential outcomes of testing. It isn't just about handing over a form to sign; it's about dialogue, understanding, and being open to answer questions and clarify doubts. These guidelines make sure that patients know exactly what their results might mean and how they could affect their lives (Roberts et al., 2020).

These standards created an environment where people feel more comfortable and secure in seeking genetic information. Without such guidelines, there could be confusion or even misuse of sensitive genetic data. Transparency ensures that patients and healthcare providers are aware of the processes and implications of genetic testing.

Nancy also believed that people needed to know about the importance of this type of study. Thus, she initiated efforts to educate the general public and the medical community on genetic counseling. These campaigns were designed to demystify genetic testing and explain it in more accessible language. This helped to reduce the misconceptions and fears associated with genetic conditions.

Nancy showed us how important it is to explore and think about ethics in science. Her journey, starting with the study of Huntington's disease in Venezuela, highlights the power of empathy and respect in research. She demonstrated that scientific progress must always be balanced with ethical responsibility, proving that it's possible to make a difference while being kind and thoughtful.

Having a progressive fatal disease such as Huntington's is significantly different from living with a stable disability. Still, it does not preclude a worthwhile life, with the resources and support that can make this possible. Those of us at risk for this disease have learned to value our precarious relationship to the world, and the insights that it has given us. –Nancy Wexler

Chapter 12:

Anne McLaren—Fertility and Embryology Expert

Anne McLaren undertook pivotal work in fertility and embryology. Her remarkable breakthroughs have transformed our understanding of human reproduction. She investigated the complexities of genetic mechanisms, initiated a revolution in fertility treatments, and advanced the field of embryology. She explored the processes that govern mammalian development to find the key to enhancing fertility.

Groundbreaking Research in Mammalian Genetics

Anne McLaren was a true pioneer in genetic mechanisms in mammalian development. In the 1950s, while at the Royal Veterinary College, Anne coauthored a groundbreaking paper that documented the successful birth of mice developed in vitro. This proved that it was possible to develop embryos outside the mother's body, setting the stage for human in vitro fertilization (IVF). This discovery eventually led to the birth of the first IVF baby, Louise Brown, 20 years later (The Royal Society, n.d.).

To understand reproduction, Anne studied how mammal embryos evolved within the mother's womb. When she was able to isolate and study the genetic mechanisms, she enhanced her scientific comprehension of how embryos grow and develop. Shortly afterward, Anne and her team were able to develop effective fertility treatments to help people who wanted to become parents but couldn't due to biological conditions. Her research, therefore, became a cornerstone upon which future reproductive technologies were built (Delaine, 2020).

Her work also significantly impacted future research in reproductive technology, influencing studies on infertility that continue to this day. Beyond the progress in the realm of biology, her efforts have touched countless lives by opening the door to parenthood for those experiencing infertility issues.

First Female Officer of the Royal Society

Anne made her discoveries while she was the director of the Medical Research Council's Mammalian Development Unit at University College London from 1974 to 1992. Following her time at University College London, McLaren further advanced her research as an investigator at the Wellcome Cancer Research Institute, which later became the Gurdon Institute at the University of Cambridge. Here, she continued to unravel the complexities of mammalian development while also engaging with the broader implications of her work, especially regarding ethical considerations.

One of McLaren's most notable qualities was her willingness to confront the ethical dilemmas associated with emerging reproductive technologies. As assisted reproductive technologies such as IVF became more prevalent, questions surrounding preimplantation genetic diagnosis and chimeric stem cell research emerged. Anne actively participated in these discussions, emphasizing the need for thoughtful consideration of the ethical implications tied to scientific advancements.

Her involvement with the Warnock Committee, established in response to the birth of Louise Brown, the first baby conceived through IVF, exemplifies her commitment to ethical discourse. She was actively involved in shaping policy recommendations regarding the regulation of human fertilization and embryology. Her insights contributed to establishing responsible frameworks that governed the use of reproductive technologies in society.

Anne didn't just stop at being an inspiring figurehead; she actively advocated for women's presence and success in science, emphasizing the importance of support systems. Through her efforts, the scientific community began to acknowledge and address the challenges faced by women, thereby underscoring the strides they'd made in traditionally male-dominated fields.

One of the lasting impacts of McLaren's legacy came through her dedication to mentoring young female scientists. She understood the transformative power of nurturing talent and providing guidance to those starting their careers. Her mentorship style emphasized collaboration, encouragement, and growth, which significantly contributed to building a supportive and empowering environment. By investing time into mentoring, McLaren ensured that her mentees were well-equipped to tackle challenges and make meaningful contributions to the scientific community.

McLaren's advocacy extended well beyond British borders, particularly during the Cold War era when she made frequent trips to the USSR. There, she established connections with scientists and strengthened ties with Soviet science academies, often smuggling cash to support financially struggling researchers. Her commitment to science was also evident in her efforts to promote research in developing countries, including Cuba, China, and India, where she worked to foster collaborations with the UK.

However, her political beliefs complicated her travels. As an active member of the Communist Party of Great Britain, McLaren faced restrictions that prevented her from visiting the United States for much of her career. Despite these challenges, her scientific achievements were widely recognized. In 1975, she became a Fellow of the Royal Society, and she went on to become the first female officer in this esteemed organization, first as foreign secretary and later as vice president. She also held the presidency of the British Association for the Advancement of Science and the Association for Women in Science and Engineering (AWISE), of which she was a founder member.

Her exemplary career culminated in 2002 with the Japan Prize, akin to the Nobel Prize, for her work in mammalian embryonic development. In 1993, she was made a Dame of the British Empire, although her response was anything but traditional. She replied: "Oh bother, I'm really rather busy at the moment, but thank you anyway" (Delaine, 2020, para. 13).

Although she typically avoided titles, McLaren specifically dismissed "Dame" because it seemed old-fashioned and lacked the flair associated with the male title "Sir." Consequently, her research team often referred to her as "Sir Anne."

When I see the appalling problems that other women are having to face, not only in this country but all over the world, the contrasts with my own life strikes [sic] *me very forcibly. I don't do much for AWISE; likewise AWISE itself can't do much; but unless we all do what we can, how will things ever get better?*
–Anne McLaren

Chapter 13:

Mary Edwards Walker—The Medal of Honor Surgeon

Mary Edwards Walker was awarded the Medal of Honor, a remarkable achievement in military history that symbolized a significant step forward in the fight for women's rights. At a time when societal norms heavily restricted women's roles, Mary courageously defied expectations by serving as a contract surgeon for the Union Army during the Civil War. Her bravery and dedication saved countless lives on dangerous battlefields.

Her extraordinary experiences during the Civil War, including treating wounded soldiers and enduring capture by Confederate forces, illustrate her steadfast commitment to equality and justice.

Only Woman to Receive the Medal of Honor

Mary Edwards Walker was the first and only woman to receive the Medal of Honor. As the highest military decoration, the Medal of Honor represents extraordinary acts of valor. It is given to recognize bravery and heroism during active combat.

During the American Civil War, Mary was awarded the Medal of Honor for her service as a contract surgeon for the Union Army, where she treated wounded soldiers on some of the most perilous battlefields. This role was traditionally reserved for men. In 1861, she became a contract surgeon, joining the 52nd Ohio Volunteer Infantry and working tirelessly to care for wounded soldiers on the battlefield, often in dangerous conditions.

Mary served primarily as a surgeon rather than as a combatant in specific battles. However, she was involved in various military campaigns and was present at several key locations during the Civil War. Notably, she worked in the field at the First Battle of Bull Run in 1861, where she faced the grim realities of war, treating wounded soldiers. Her most significant service included working at hospitals and on the battlefield, which included accompanying the Army of the Potomac during various campaigns, such as the Peninsular Campaign in 1862. Walker's role was crucial in providing medical care, and she often traveled with the army, attending to wounded troops wherever she was needed. While she didn't fight in battles in the traditional sense, her presence on the front lines and her contributions to medical care during the war greatly impacted the lives of many soldiers.

Her recognition didn't come without controversy. Many questioned whether a woman could truly embody the valor typically associated with this honor. They considered that her role during the war wasn't enough to deserve the award. This is a reflection of the gender prejudices at the time.

Despite these challenges, Mary remained undeterred. She often found herself close to battle lines, tending to soldiers amid the chaos and danger of war. But taking care of the wounded wasn't her only feat. She was captured by Confederate forces in 1864 when she was in Confederate territory near Atlanta, Georgia.

During her captivity, Mary faced significant challenges, including harsh conditions and the stigma associated with her gender. She was held for several months, and during this time she continued to advocate for her fellow prisoners and maintained her resolve. In response to her capture and the poor treatment of Union soldiers, efforts were made to secure her release.

After a few months in captivity, she was eventually exchanged for a Confederate prisoner as part of a prisoner exchange agreement. Following her release, she continued her work and remained dedicated to the Union cause, contributing to medical efforts until the end of the war.

Although her medal was later revoked due to changes in the eligibility criteria, President Jimmy Carter reinstated it posthumously in 1977, acknowledging Mary's rightful place in history as the only woman to receive this revered accolade.

Advocating for Women's Dress Reform

Mary also boldly stood at the forefront of the dress reform movement, which aimed for liberation from the restrictive clothing norms of the 19th century. At that time, women's clothes included tight corsets and voluminous skirts, which were often uncomfortable and limited freedom of movement. Mary recognized how these fashion choices restricted women physically and symbolically. It was a way to limit what women could do.

Instead of dresses, Mary chose to wear trousers and jackets. She believed that women had the right and power to decide what they wore. Moreover, her medical background provided her with insights into the adverse health effects of corsets, which compressed the internal organs. Her message wasn't only against social prejudices but also about the importance of women's health and autonomy over their bodies.

People reacted in varied ways when they saw Mary walking through the streets in jeans. While some saw her as a disruptor who defied social norms, others admired her courage and conviction. Walker faced arrest several times for wearing "men's clothing," as it was considered scandalous for a woman. On one occasion, she proudly marched in her "man's" clothes through the streets of New York City, ignoring the jeers and scorn from passersby.

Her fight wasn't about fashion. She argued that liberating attire could empower women, giving them the freedom to participate more fully in public life, work, and physical activities. Her ideas would later contribute to the evolution of women's fashion into styles based on utility and comfort.

Through her pioneering achievements in military medicine and her passionate advocacy for women's dress reform, Mary continuously broke barriers and challenged societal norms. Her receipt of the Medal of Honor, despite being surrounded by controversy, paved the way for important discussions about women's roles both in the military and beyond.

Let the generations know that women in uniform also guaranteed their freedom.
–Mary Edwards Walker

Chapter 14:

Gertrude Elion—Innovative Drug Developer

Gertrude B. Elion's passion for science drove her to break new ground in drug development, creating medications that have transformed lives and offered hope to countless patients around the globe. Her work transcended traditional methods, leading to discoveries that changed how we understand and treat some of the most challenging diseases. An influential biochemist and pharmacologist, her groundbreaking work in drug development earned her a place among the great scientists of her time.

Against All Odds

Born on January 23, 1918, in New York City, Elion faced numerous challenges in pursuing her education and career due to the pervasive gender biases of her era.

Gertrude's early life was profoundly shaped by her close relationship with her grandfather, who had emigrated from Russia when she was just three years old. This bond left an indelible mark on her, and by the age of 15 she faced the emotional turmoil of witnessing his painful demise from stomach cancer. This heart-wrenching experience greatly influenced her decision to pursue a career in science, specifically pharmacology, driven by a desire to alleviate suffering through medical advancements.

However, her aspirations faced a significant setback when the stock market crash of 1929 led to her family's bankruptcy, casting doubt on her future. Despite excelling academically and securing a place at Hunter College—one of the few free institutions available—Elion encountered challenges with finances post-graduation.

She aspired to continue her education in graduate school but quickly realized that fellowships were scarce and rarely awarded to women, particularly during the economic hardships of the Great Depression. At just 19 and armed with a degree in chemistry, she found herself navigating a challenging job market. Elion took on various roles, including secretary, chemistry teacher, and unpaid assistant in a laboratory, determined to gain experience in her field. Her perseverance eventually paid off when World War II led to a shortage of male chemists, creating opportunities for women. This shift in demand allowed Elion to secure a position in a laboratory, marking the beginning of her groundbreaking career in pharmaceuticals and paving the way for her future innovations in drug development (*Gertrude B. Elion*, n.d.).

One of the most interesting aspects of Elion's life is her academic journey. After earning a bachelor's degree from Hunter College, she pursued graduate studies at New York University. However, she faced challenges in securing a PhD program, partly due to gender discrimination, and instead began working in a laboratory at the age of 23, where she gained invaluable research experience.

Developing Treatments for Leukemia and Organ Rejection

Gertrude revolutionized drug discovery through rational drug design. Her innovative process involved targeting specific differences between normal cells and pathogens or cancer cells. She worked with her colleague, George Hitchings. Together, they moved away from the traditional trial-and-error approach and focused on understanding the biochemical processes of diseases (*Gertrude B. Elion*, n.d.).

Early in her career, she developed acyclovir, the first effective antiviral drug for treating herpes simplex virus infections. Approved by the U.S. Food and Drug Administration in 1981, acyclovir revolutionized the management of herpesvirus infections and greatly reduced the severity and duration of outbreaks, providing relief for millions of patients worldwide.

One of her most important contributions was her breakthrough leukemia treatment. In the mid-20th century, leukemia was almost invariably fatal, particularly when it affected children. Gertrude, however, was determined to alter that bleak outlook. She worked on drugs like 6-mercaptopurine (6-MP), which helped treat childhood leukemia. These drugs stopped leukemia cells from making DNA, preventing them from growing (*Gertrude B. Elion*, n.d.).

She also played a key role in developing mercaptopurine, a drug used in the treatment of acute lymphoblastic leukemia and other cancers. Approved in the 1950s, mercaptopurine became one of the standard treatments for childhood leukemia, greatly improving survival rates for affected patients. Elion's important work led to much higher survival rates; children who had little hope could now go into remission and live longer, healthier lives.

Elion didn't stop at just improving cancer treatments. She also investigated the field of immunosuppressive drugs and made significant strides in transplant medicine. Before her innovations, organ rejection was a major hurdle in transplants, often leading to the failure of these critical procedures. However, with the discovery of azathioprine, Gertrude opened new doors for transplant patients. This drug effectively suppressed the body's natural defense mechanism against foreign organs, and this allowed successful transplantation. The body didn't reject the new organ any longer. As a result, countless individuals received a second chance at life through organ transplants.

Gertrude's relentless pursuit of knowledge led her to publish over 225 scientific papers, each contributing to our understanding of disease mechanisms and treatment strategies.

Nobel Prize in Physiology

In recognition of her extraordinary contributions to medicine, Elion was awarded numerous accolades throughout her career. In 1988, she, along with Hitchings and Sir James Black, was awarded the Nobel Prize in Physiology or Medicine. Elion was also elected to the National Academy of Sciences and received the National Medal of Science.

Gertrude's path to the Nobel Prize was built on challenges and perseverance. She faced abundant obstacles, ranging from discrimination in academia to scant financial support. Early in her career, she experienced numerous rejections from graduate schools (Memorial Sloan Kettering Cancer Center, n.d.).

Beyond her scientific achievements, Elion was a trailblazer for women in science. She served as a mentor to many young scientists, encouraging them to pursue their passions and break barriers in the field.

Gertrude Elion passed away on February 3, 2019, leaving a lasting legacy as a pioneer in pharmacology and a role model for future generations of women in STEM. From her groundbreaking development of treatments for leukemia, dramatically shifting survival rates for children, to her innovations in transplant medicine, Gertrude paved new paths with her inventive spirit.

Nobody... took me seriously. They wondered why in the world I wanted to be a chemist when no women were doing that. The world was not waiting for me.
–Gertrude B. Elion

Chapter 15:

Frances Oldham Kelsey—

Protecting Public Health

Frances Oldham Kelsey's story unfolds against the backdrop of the 1960s, when the medical community was facing new challenges in drug regulation. Kelsey, armed with scientific training and strong ethical convictions, entered this world.

She wouldn't give in to pressure from drug companies that wanted to sell their products quickly. Instead, Kelsey insisted on thorough testing and clear evidence of safety, showing the need to protect public health even when facing challenges. Her commitment saved many lives and helped create stricter rules for approving drugs, which still influence healthcare today.

Kelsey's Influence on Drug Safety Regulations

Born on July 24, 1914, in Cobourg, Ontario, Canada, Kelsey showed early academic promise. She earned her Bachelor of Arts degree from McGill University and went on to receive her Doctor of Medicine from the University of Chicago in 1950. Her strong educational foundation in both pharmacology and medicine would later inform her groundbreaking work.

In the early 1960s, a drug named thalidomide became an alarming symbol of inadequate drug safety testing. Approved in many countries as a remedy for morning sickness in pregnant women, it tragically resulted in severe birth defects affecting over 10,000 children worldwide.

This catastrophe highlighted a major flaw: the lack of stringent drug approval processes.

Kelsey was a relatively new employee at the U.S. Food and Drug Administration (FDA) when she learned about thalidomide. Pharmaceutical companies were pressing to get their products into the market, but Frances was aware of the dangers and refused to give the green light without conclusive evidence of its safety. She joined other colleagues such as Helen Taussig (see Chapter 4) and worked to prevent the approval of thalidomide in the United States, sparing countless families from its devastating effects.

Frances's unwavering pursuit of safety contributed to the passage of the Kefauver–Harris Amendment in 1962. This law changed how drugs are approved in the US. Prior to the amendment, the Federal Food, Drug, and Cosmetic Act of 1938 primarily required that drugs be shown to be safe for use. The Kefauver–Harris Amendment introduced the requirement that drug manufacturers demonstrate not only safety but also efficacy before a drug could be approved for sale. This requirement marked a pivotal shift from a focus solely on safety to an emphasis on both safety and therapeutic effectiveness.

The amendment also mandated that informed consent be obtained from clinical trial participants. It required that individuals participating in drug trials be fully informed about the nature of the research, any potential risks associated with the drug, and their right to withdraw from the study at any time. This provision aimed to protect the rights and well-being of research participants.

The Kefauver–Harris Amendment also established stringent requirements for reporting adverse reactions to drugs. Manufacturers were obligated to report any serious side effects associated with their products, enhancing the monitoring of drug safety after a drug entered the market.

The amendment granted the FDA increased authority over the drug approval process, including the power to ensure compliance with the new standards. This legislative change empowered the FDA to take a more active role in overseeing clinical trials and evaluating the safety and efficacy of new drugs.

The Kefauver–Harris Amendment promoted similar regulatory reforms in other countries, establishing principles of drug safety and efficacy that remain integral to pharmaceutical regulation today.

The impact of Frances's contributions had enduring effects on public trust in pharmaceuticals. People needed to be assured that what they consumed was indeed safe. This impact is still felt today, as the FDA continues to uphold the stringent measures she championed.

Recognition and Legacy of Frances Oldham Kelsey

For her courageous stand against thalidomide, Kelsey received numerous accolades, including the President's Award for Distinguished Federal Civilian Service in 1962. This award was given to individuals who have made extraordinary contributions to public welfare.

After receiving the award, Frances remained focused on what truly mattered to her: patient welfare. Her humility in accepting the award highlighted her dedication to protecting lives over seeking personal recognition. She graciously accepted the honor while redirecting attention back to the importance of rigorous drug testing and safety.

The Federal Civil Service Award helped her cause gain more attention and attract more supporters for safer medicine practices. With more people aware of the issue, Kelsey was able to influence the process of making policies, showing how important individual recognition can be in creating social change.

Public recognition, like the award Kelsey received, does more than praise previous actions; it encourages future efforts. Her award inspired healthcare professionals everywhere, highlighting the need for integrity and support for safe practices. Healthcare professionals were reminded of their duty to prioritize patient safety above all else, fostering a culture where ethical considerations became paramount.

After retiring, Kelsey remained involved in public health issues and continued to speak on matters related to drug safety. She was recognized in various forums, including the 2011 documentary *The Drug That Changed the World*, which highlighted her contributions and the importance of ethical practices in pharmacology.

Frances Oldham Kelsey passed away on August 7, 2015, but her legacy as a pioneer in drug safety and public health advocacy remains influential and inspirational, highlighting the importance of vigilance in protecting public health from pharmaceutical risks.

Emphasizing the importance of rigorous testing, Frances ensured that the safety of countless individuals was prioritized over economic interests, preventing tragedies like thalidomide from unfolding in the US. Her actions showcased the power of scientific integrity and taught us the importance of standing firm in our values, even when faced with immense pressure.

When a woman took a job in those days, she was made feel as if she was depriving a man of the ability to support his wife and child. But my professor said: "Don't be stupid. Accept the job, sign your name and put 'Miss' in brackets afterward."
–Frances Oldham Kelsey

Chapter 16:

Jane Cooke Wright—Chemotherapy Innovator

Jane Cooke Wright's work in chemotherapy was an innovative approach to cancer treatment. She focused on understanding how different drugs interact with cancer cells to enable treatments to be tailored to individual needs, ultimately changing the medical landscape. This chapter invites you to discover the incredible ways in which Wright's dedication led to significant advancements in chemotherapy, forever altering how we fight against this challenging disease.

Pioneering Use of Human Tissue Cultures for Drug Testing

Jane Cooke Wright was a remarkable doctor and scientist who made significant contributions to medicine, especially in the field of cancer research. Born in 1919, she grew up in a family that valued education. Her father was a doctor and her mother was a social worker, which inspired her to pursue a career in medicine. Wright attended Smith College, where she studied medical sciences, and later graduated from the New York Medical College in 1945. She became one of the first women to break through the barriers in the medical field, proving that women could excel in science and medicine just like men.

One of her most significant contributions was developing human tissue cultures to accurately predict how patients might respond to chemotherapy drugs. Before this advancement, doctors could only guess how a patient's body might react to treatment, leading to trials that weren't always successful. By using tissue cultures from patients, Wright created a method that allowed physicians to get an idea of the likely effectiveness of different drugs.

Thanks to her idea, it was possible to personalize treatments, which significantly increased success rates and saved more people's lives. Wright also played a crucial role in using combination chemotherapy. This means using more than one drug at a time to attack cancer cells from different angles, making it harder for the cancer to survive. Her research helped improve survival rates for many patients with leukemia and other types of cancer (Elliott, 2016).

Another innovative approach was Jane's focus on improving drug efficacy. She demonstrated how certain chemotherapy drugs could be more effective against particular types of cancer. This targeted approach meant that instead of using broad-spectrum drugs on all patients, doctors could tailor treatment plans to match the specific cancers they were dealing with. This improved patient outcomes and reduced unnecessary side effects. The ability to accurately target cancer cells while sparing healthy ones has paved the way for today's targeted therapies in cancer treatment.

Wright's influence extended beyond direct patient treatment, impacting research methodologies in profound ways. Her techniques were widely adopted among researchers, who began refining these methods further to explore other complex cancer treatments. Research in oncology steered toward more personalized and data-driven approaches (Falzone et al., 2018).

The principles she established are still evident in today's treatments, including targeted therapy and immunotherapy, which have increased survival rates and quality of life for many cancer patients (Elliott, 2016).

Jane Cooke Wright had a major impact on modern cancer treatment. Without her work, advances such as monoclonal antibodies, immune checkpoint inhibitors, and personalized medicine might not exist. Her innovative ideas and commitment to improving care for cancer patients have significantly affected the medical field, showing how one dedicated scientist can help save lives.

First African American Woman Elected as a Fellow of the New York Academy of Medicine

One of Wright's most distinguished accomplishments was her participation as a fellow in prominent early research programs. This fellowship showcased her groundbreaking work in cancer research and positioned her as an advocate for gender inclusivity within scientific circles.

Her advocacy for diversity had an immense influence on medical institutions. Her contributions to medicine proved the need for equal opportunities in research environments. Wright's career unfolded during a transformational period in American history, marked by milestones like the signing of the Civil Rights Act of 1964. In this context, she cofounded the American Society for Clinical Oncology alongside six male colleagues, defying the norms of the time.

Jane dedicated herself to helping patients, training new doctors, and advocating for more research in cancer. She served as the first female director of the cancer research department at New York Medical College and was involved in various health organizations.

Jane consistently emphasized the importance of personalized patient care. She believed that each cancer patient had a unique story and that understanding their individual experiences was crucial in providing effective treatment. She taught medical students to listen carefully to their patients, encouraging them to ask questions and understand the emotional struggles patients faced. Many of her students went on to adopt this patient-centered approach, improving relationships between doctors and patients in their own practices.

Her work extended beyond the walls of the medical college. Jane became involved with the American Medical Women's Association, where she was a strong voice for women in medicine. She fought against the barriers that prevented women from advancing in their careers. Jane organized workshops and mentorship programs designed to inspire young women to pursue careers in healthcare. She regularly spoke at events, sharing her own experiences and encouraging aspiring doctors to follow their dreams, despite the challenges they might face in a male-dominated field.

Jane understood the emotional toll that cancer could take on patients and their families; she believed that support services were just as important as medical care. She initiated support groups within the hospital to connect patients with others facing similar challenges. These groups provided a safe space for sharing experiences and fostering hope. Jane often attended these meetings herself, offering her guidance and encouragement. Her presence helped build a community where patients felt understood and supported in their journeys.

Even with the increasing burden of cancer, Jane remained optimistic about the future. She often reflected on the progress made in treatment options and the growing number of survivors. Her unwavering belief in the power of research and education fueled her dedication. As she continued her work, Jane kept her sights set on driving further advancements in the field of oncology, knowing that every small step brought the medical community closer to finding a cure.

Jane Cooke Wright didn't just develop innovative ways to treat cancer; she altered how researchers approach treatment, making it more personal and effective. Her work with human tissue cultures gave doctors a clearer picture of how specific drugs might interact with different types of cancer, leading to treatments that were both targeted and successful. Wright's contributions have forever changed the landscape of cancer research, paving the way for modern therapies that continue to evolve today.

I know I'm a member of two minority groups, but I don't think of myself that way. Sure, a woman has to try twice as hard. But, racial prejudice? I've met very little of it. It could be I met it – and wasn't intelligent enough to recognize it.
–Jane Cooke Wright

Chapter 17:

Susan La Flesche Picotte—

Native American Medical Advocate

As the first Native American woman physician, Susan La Flesche Picotte broke barriers in a time when her people couldn't access quality healthcare. She was born into the Omaha tribe, and from a very young age she committed to transforming the health landscape of her community. Her resolve to become a doctor and serve on the Omaha Reservation laid the groundwork for reshaping public health among Native American communities.

Throughout this chapter, you'll explore Susan La Flesche Picotte's pioneering efforts to establish the first private hospital on a reservation, which stood as a beacon of hope and progress.

First Private Hospital on a Reservation

Susan La Flesche Picotte was born on June 17, 1865, on the Omaha Reservation in Nebraska. Established in the 19th century, the reservation is home to the Omaha people, a federally recognized tribe with a rich cultural heritage and history. The reservation is situated along the Missouri River and encompasses parts of Burt and Thurston counties. The reservation was created following the signing of treaties between the Omaha tribe and the United States government.

She was the daughter of a prominent Omaha chief, and her upbringing was deeply influenced by both her Native American heritage and the values of education that her parents instilled in her. Her mother Mary was a strong advocate for education, which played a significant role in shaping Susan's ambition. Growing up in a time when opportunities for women, especially women of color, were limited, Susan faced numerous challenges. Nonetheless, she was determined to pursue her education. She attended the local school on the reservation, where she excelled in her studies. Recognizing her potential, her parents encouraged her to continue her education beyond the reservation.

At the age of 14, Susan moved to Elizabeth, New Jersey, to attend a boarding school, where she further developed her academic skills. Her dedication and hard work paid off when she was accepted to the Woman's Medical College of Pennsylvania, one of the few medical schools available to women at the time. In 1889, she graduated with her medical degree, becoming the first Native American woman to earn a medical degree in the United States.

After completing her studies, Susan returned to the Omaha Reservation, where she devoted herself to improving the health and well-being of her people. Faced with a lack of medical facilities and resources, she worked tirelessly to provide healthcare to her community. She emphasized the importance of preventive care and education about health, often traveling long distances to reach those in need.

Throughout her life, Susan broke barriers and championed the rights of Native Americans, advocating for better healthcare and social reforms. Her journey from a young girl on the Omaha Reservation to a pioneering doctor exemplified her unwavering determination and commitment to her community.

Susan established the first private hospital on the Omaha Reservation, which became a fundamental resource for medical care for the people of this community. Building the hospital on the Omaha Reservation was an unprecedented move at a time when Native American communities had very limited access to quality healthcare. With modern equipment and facilities, the hospital addressed a range of health needs, making emergency care more readily available to those who needed it most.

Picotte's hospital played a vital role in improving overall health outcomes on the Omaha Reservation, alleviating many of the preventable health issues that plagued the area. For example, epidemics like smallpox had previously taken dozens of lives, and communities had few options for combating the disease. However, with the establishment of the hospital, there was a reliable source of medical intervention.

The hospital was founded in 1913 with the help and support of Picotte and community leaders, becoming the first private hospital for Native Americans in the United States. The facility aimed to address the health disparities faced by the Omaha tribe and provided a range of healthcare services, including general medical care, maternity care, and treatment for various diseases. Picotte focused on emphasizing preventive care and education, promoting healthy practices within the community.

One of the keys to her success was her ability to involve the community in health education. Local residents participated in various health education initiatives, which empowered them with the knowledge necessary to take charge of their health. This involvement fostered a sense of trust and collaboration between the hospital staff and members of the community.

Moreover, the hospital stood as a symbol of hope and empowerment for Native American communities across the nation. Susan's achievements inspired other communities to pursue their healthcare rights. She spread a powerful message: Indigenous people could define their destinies and improve their conditions through perseverance and a collective effort.

Promoting Vaccination and Hygiene Education

Susan was the first Native American woman physician and a pioneer in public health and education. Her efforts focused on disease prevention, an approach that blended modern medical practices with traditional wisdom.

One of her most notable contributions was her vigor in promoting vaccination efforts. During her time, outbreaks of infectious diseases like smallpox and influenza were terrible threats to Native American communities. Picotte understood that prevention could safeguard health and worked to educate her community on the benefits of vaccinations.

By organizing health campaigns and dispelling myths surrounding vaccines, she managed to significantly reduce disease occurrence within the Omaha Reservation. Her strategy involved engaging community members through talks and distributing easily understandable pamphlets. The campaigns had positive results and resulted in many more people going to the hospital for vaccinations (Centers for Disease Control and Prevention, 2024).

In addition to promoting vaccination, Picotte also highlighted the importance of hygiene to prevent the spread of infections. She organized workshops with people in the community to teach them essential hygiene practices such as handwashing, proper waste disposal, and food safety.

Furthermore, Picotte understood the importance of collaboration in expanding healthcare outreach. She partnered with local tribal leaders and national health organizations to bring the necessary resources and expertise to her community. For instance, she aimed to integrate traditional wisdom with Western medical techniques. As a result, a strong culture of health awareness emerged in the Omaha Reservation and beyond.

Her advocacy cultivated a community environment where people felt empowered to take charge of their own health, and her legacy laid the groundwork for subsequent generations to continue advancing the health of Native American communities. Many young women from her tribe pursued careers in medicine and public health, motivated by Picotte's example of dedication and resilience.

Susan La Flesche Picotte transformed healthcare access for Native American communities by building the first private hospital on the Omaha Reservation. Her dedication to promoting vaccination and hygiene education was key to creating healthier living conditions.

I am a dreamer who dreams, sees visions, and listens always to the still, small voice. I am a trail-blazer. –Susan La Flesche Picotte

Chapter 18:

Lucille Teasdale-Corti—Compassion in Conflict Zones

Lucille Teasdale-Corti's impact in Uganda began with her commitment to building a healthcare foundation, even though the country was going through the challenges of conflict and scarcity. Lucille had a dream of establishing a hospital in the city of Gulu and, eventually, it transformed from vision to reality. Through her dedication, she provided immediate medical care and laid down a healthcare framework designed to endure through time and turmoil.

Establishing a Major Hospital in Gulu, Uganda

Lucille Teasdale-Corti's story started when she arrived in Uganda, a country facing many problems due to war and poverty. She was from Canada but left after completing her medical education. Lucille arrived in Uganda in 1962, intending to work as a volunteer surgeon at the Teba Hospital in the remote region of Kumi. By that time, the country was in the middle of a political and social crisis.

She established Gulu Hospital, which became more than just a place for medical care—it served as a symbol of hope for many people. She wanted to go beyond simply providing quick help; she aimed to create a strong healthcare system that could handle future challenges.

Teasdale-Corti recognized early on that founding a hospital in such a turbulent environment required more than just medical expertise. It demanded courage, leadership, and a deep understanding of the community's needs. She envisioned a facility that would not only treat patients but also educate the local population ("Malaria Is Once Again Killing in Uganda," 2015).

Initially, Teasdale-Corti faced numerous challenges, including a lack of medical supplies and infrastructure. Despite these obstacles, she quickly gained a reputation for her skill and compassion. Over the years, she performed thousands of surgeries and treated countless patients, often working long hours under difficult conditions. Her commitment to the community extended beyond the operating room; she was instrumental in training local medical staff and improving healthcare practices.

The political landscape in Uganda became increasingly tumultuous after the rise of Idi Amin in 1971, leading to widespread violence and chaos. Many healthcare professionals left the country, but Teasdale-Corti remained steadfast in her mission. During this time, she was known to risk her own safety to provide care to those in need, including victims of torture and violence.

She understood the power of collaboration, especially with the local community. She ensured that solutions were culturally appropriate and sustainable. Women, in particular, played a significant role in this ecosystem. She initiated programs that empowered women to become healthcare advocates in their communities.

These collaborative efforts transformed Gulu Hospital into a point of reference for healthcare in the region. Teasdale-Corti cultivated an environment of mutual respect and learning. Her approach exemplified the importance of inclusive healthcare models where the community is an active participant in health-related decisions.

Teasdale-Corti's work at Gulu Hospital had a long-lasting impact. The hospital continues to serve communities in the region, adapting to modern challenges while preserving the foundational principles laid by Teasdale.

Implementing Surgical Programs Under Difficult Conditions

Imagine handling surgeries with scarce resources and equipment, yet still finding ways to save lives and improve healthcare standards. This wasn't an ordinary feat. However, Teasdale-Corti perfected techniques that made it possible to conduct critical operations with whatever was available. It required creativity, adaptability, and a deep understanding of how to make the most of every resource. For instance, she might use basic tools to perform sophisticated procedures. She didn't have the chance to buy or otherwise get hold of medical supplies, but she still wanted to save people's lives. So, she managed to find resources wherever she could.

Handling emergency surgeries became another area where she shone. The situations she experienced were often tense, with life-or-death scenarios unfolding rapidly. Yet she managed these high-stress environments with calmness and professionalism. Imagine performing a delicate operation with the sounds of gunshots and screams outside. Such conditions could easily frazzle even the most experienced surgeon. However, Lucille's ability to maintain focus and composure demonstrated her professionalism in the medical field. Her example taught others that staying calm allows for better decision-making.

The success of her surgical programs had a profound impact on the whole community, not only on the people who underwent surgery. It instilled trust in doctors in a context where everybody was afraid and suspicious, so building trust was no small task. Initially, the community may have been skeptical, particularly with ongoing conflicts affecting their daily lives. But as more people were healed after Lucille's surgeries, the reputation of healthcare services improved. Then, people felt more confident to seek healthcare. This trust was pivotal because it encouraged proactive healthcare engagement among community members, thereby improving overall health outcomes.

Furthermore, Teasdale-Corti's efforts showcased the power of determination. She demonstrated how improving surgical care isn't solely about technology but also about using your wits and adaptability to solve problems. Similarly, her commitment to training local healthcare providers teaches us the significance of investing in people. It shows that mentorship and knowledge sharing are vital for creating systems capable of standing the test of time and overcoming challenges.

Lucille Teasdale-Corti built a hospital and created a place of hope and learning. By involving the local community, especially women, she ensured that everyone had a role in improving healthcare. This approach helped build trust and made sure that health services would continue to grow and improve even after she was gone.

If you are convinced by what you are doing, if you truly believe in it, then you stay. There is no other way. –Lucille Teasdale-Corti

Chapter 19:

Barbara McClintock—A Pioneer in Genetics

Barbara McClintock stands as a celebrated figure in genetics, renowned for her groundbreaking discoveries despite facing numerous challenges throughout her life. We'll discuss how her upbringing played a pivotal role in shaping her as a scientist and examine the hurdles she faced while studying in predominantly male environments. Barbara's early experiences show us how her remarkable resolve and intellect set her on a path toward making revolutionary contributions to genetics.

Early Life and Academic Challenges

Barbara McClintock was born in 1902, in Hartford, Connecticut. Her early years were marked by a burgeoning curiosity about the world around her—an enthusiasm that was warmly encouraged by her family, especially her mother.

This supportive environment allowed Barbara to maintain her passion for scientific pursuits, even though societal norms during her youth often discouraged women from entering such fields. Throughout her educational journey, Barbara navigated a landscape dominated by male counterparts, often finding herself at odds with prevailing gender biases. Yet her determination was unwavering. She pushed forward into academia, enrolling in Cornell University, where she was one of the few women pursuing studies in agricultural and plant sciences. It was here that she developed the resilience and skills necessary to contribute significantly to science.

Throughout her academic career, Barbara encountered discrimination that could have easily discouraged a less determined individual. For instance, it wasn't uncommon for Barbara to be excluded from discussions or experiments simply because of her gender. Such instances of bias only seemed to fortify her determination to succeed. Instead of being disheartened by these experiences, Barbara used them as fuel for her perseverance (*Women's History Month—Barbara McClintock*, 2014).

While navigating this challenging environment, Barbara also benefited from the mentorship of several key figures who recognized her immense potential. Among her mentors were leading scientists who valued intellect over social norms and championed her capabilities regardless of the prevailing biases. Their guidance and belief in her abilities provided essential support systems, helping her advance in her studies and research endeavors. These mentors served as allies who helped Barbara forge a path in genetics, giving her the encouragement needed to persist in a field that was resistant to her presence.

Barbara's time at Cornell was marked by both triumphs and tests. During her graduate studies, she continued to excel academically, earning her BS in 1923, her MA in 1925, and her PhD in 1927. While institutional gender barriers persisted, Barbara found comfort in the lab, where her ideas and creativity could flourish. Here, she began to form the foundation for her future groundbreaking work.

The environment at Cornell, while challenging, also offered fertile ground for Barbara's development as a scientist. Engaging deeply with her peers and professors, Barbara pushed the boundaries of what was considered possible in plant genetics. These experiences instilled in her a lifelong appreciation for hands-on research and critical thinking (*4th Medical Trip*, 2024).

Breakthrough Discoveries and Legacy

Barbara's major scientific contributions have left a lasting impact. One of her most groundbreaking achievements was the discovery of transposable elements, often called "jumping genes." This revolutionary concept fundamentally transformed our understanding of genetics.

Genes are the basic units of heredity in living organisms. They are segments of DNA that contain the instructions for building proteins, which perform various functions in the body. Each gene has a specific location on a chromosome and can influence traits such as eye color, hair type, and susceptibility to certain diseases. Genes are inherited by offspring from their parents, and variations in these genes contribute to the diversity of traits within a species.

Transposable elements are sequences of DNA that can change their position within the genome, thus altering gene expression and function. Previously, genetic research focused on the idea that genes were fixed in their locations on chromosomes. McClintock's discovery of these mobile genetic elements challenged this notion. She demonstrated that genes could indeed move from one location to another within the genome. This movement could cause mutations and affect how other genes are expressed.

Her work with maize, a crop plant, was crucial. At the Carnegie Institution for Science, her research with maize revealed that certain chromosomal changes could lead to variations in the plant's pigmentation. By identifying these changes, she was able to demonstrate how transposable elements contributed to genetic diversity. Her meticulous observations and innovative experiments showed that these elements could be responsible for color variations in maize kernels. The implications of her findings were vast, suggesting that genetic material was not static but dynamic.

Despite the significance of her discoveries, the initial reactions from the scientific community were tepid. During McClintock's time, genetics was dominated by more traditional views, and the idea of moving genes seemed too radical for many scientists to comprehend or accept. Consequently, her work was met with skepticism and, at times, outright dismissal. Some researchers found her ideas difficult to understand because they challenged established beliefs.

However, McClintock stood firm. Her perseverance and faith in her findings eventually paid off. The subsequent discovery of similar genetic elements in other organisms validated her results. It wasn't until decades later in the 1980s, when molecular biologists began isolating transposable elements in bacteria and other organisms, that her pioneering work gained recognition.

In 1983, McClintock was awarded the Nobel Prize in Physiology or Medicine, marking an overdue acknowledgment of her contribution. Her acceptance of the prize was marked by humility and grace; she poignantly stated, "If you know you are on the right track, if you have this inner knowledge, then nobody can turn you off... no matter what they say" (*Barbara McClintock*, n.d., para 17).

The impact of McClintock's discoveries extends far beyond her lifetime. Today, the understanding of transposable elements informs numerous areas of modern genetic research, including cancer studies. The jumping genes can play roles in genomic instability and in biotechnology applications involving genetic engineering. Her work laid the groundwork for exploring complex genetic behaviors, influencing how scientists manipulate and study genetic material in various species.

Barbara McClintock's discovery of transposable elements was a game-changer, shaking up the field of genetic research and paving the way for new ideas. Her commitment shone through, eventually earning her a Nobel Prize. But her impact reaches far beyond awards.

I never thought of stopping, and I just hated sleeping. I can't imagine having a better life. –Barbara McClintock

Chapter 20:

Flossie Wong-Staal—A Trailblazer in Virology

Flossie Wong-Staal had an inquisitive mind that led her to question everything around her from a young age, sparking her interest in understanding diseases and their impact on people. This chapter unravels how Flossie's early environment and education laid the groundwork for her future achievements.

Let's explore her groundbreaking work in HIV/AIDS research, detailing how her contributions transformed our understanding of the virus and influenced public health policies worldwide.

Early Life and Challenges Faced

Flossie Wong-Staal's journey began in Hong Kong, where she was born Yee Ching Wong in 1946. Her early environment played a significant role in shaping her curiosity and determination, qualities that would later fuel her groundbreaking contributions to virology.

Despite living in a time when girls were often not encouraged to pursue scientific careers, her parents broke tradition by enrolling her in an English-language Catholic school. This decision proved pivotal in Flossie's life, providing her with the foundation needed to excel academically, especially in science and mathematics. Her teachers quickly recognized her inquisitive nature and desire to go beyond just learning facts, encouraging her to ask "why?" questions about the world around her.

From a young age, Flossie was very interested in understanding disease outbreaks within her community. She was fascinated by why certain individuals fell ill while others remained healthy. This childhood curiosity laid the groundwork for her future career as a virologist.

At the age of 18, Flossie's life took a dramatic turn when she decided to leave Hong Kong for the United States to further her education. This move was both bold and daunting—she was stepping into a foreign land, where she would be unfamiliar with the language and cultural nuances. However, she embraced this challenge head-on. She arrived at the University of California, Los Angeles (UCLA) in 1965, adopting the name "Flossie" on the advice of her English teacher back in Hong Kong.

During her time at UCLA, Flossie's intellectual prowess became increasingly evident. She earned her PhD in molecular biology in 1972—a remarkable achievement considering that fewer than 4% of doctoral degrees in sciences were awarded to non-White women at that time. Her academic success didn't come easily, as she had to navigate the complexities of being a woman immigrant in a predominantly male field.

Groundbreaking Research and Legacy

In 1973, Wong-Staal started a postdoctoral position at the Laboratory of Tumor Cell Biology, led by renowned biomedical researcher Robert C. Gallo, at the National Cancer Institute in Bethesda, Maryland. Within a few years, she rose to the role of section chief and, over the following decade, contributed to more than 100 research articles in scientific journals. When the AIDS epidemic surfaced in the early 1980s, this lab redirected its efforts to unraveling the mysteries of this emerging disease.

In the early 1980s, the world was going through a time of great confusion and fear surrounding AIDS. Wong-Staal was part of the team that made the monumental discovery identifying HIV as the cause of the disease.

Her work transformed scientific understanding and paved the way for major advancements in molecular biology.

During this critical period, Wong-Staal and her colleagues delved into the complexities of HIV, a retrovirus that evades the immune system with remarkable genetic diversity (Kenyon, 2020). Her expertise in cloning the virus in 1985 allowed scientists to unravel its genetic code, a significant step toward understanding how HIV operates and eludes the body's defenses. This breakthrough was instrumental in developing tests to detect HIV in blood samples, leading to more effective treatment strategies and saving countless lives globally (StemBot, 2022).

To comprehend the magnitude of the challenge faced by researchers studying HIV, envision the arduous task of locating a tiny needle in an ever-shifting haystack, where the needle is not only elusive but continuously morphing. HIV is a master of disguise, adept at changing its appearance rapidly, which complicates efforts to understand its structure and behavior. This constant mutation presents a significant barrier to developing effective treatments and vaccines, as each variation can potentially evade the immune response triggered by previous infections.

Amid this complexity, Wong-Staal's groundbreaking work in 1985 marked a pivotal moment in HIV research. By becoming the first scientist to clone the virus, she effectively created a "snapshot" of HIV that provided a tangible sample for investigation. This achievement enabled researchers to examine the genetic and biochemical characteristics of the virus in unprecedented detail.

Wong-Staal's contribution not only advanced the understanding of HIV but also laid the groundwork for the development of diagnostic tools and therapeutic strategies. Her work exemplifies the perseverance and innovation required to tackle one of the most formidable public health challenges of our time, propelling HIV research into a new era.

The discoveries initiated by Wong-Staal had profound implications beyond the laboratory. They revolutionized public health policies worldwide, shaping the way in which governments and healthcare organizations approached HIV/AIDS prevention and treatment. Thanks to her work, antiretroviral therapies became a reality, transforming HIV from a fatal diagnosis into a manageable chronic condition. The ability to test for HIV antibodies enabled early detection, which was crucial for controlling its spread. Her contributions also improved people's potential to be treated and have a better quality of life.

Beyond the lab, Flossie's influence expanded as she received numerous accolades for her contributions to science. These honors offered her a platform to advocate for greater awareness of HIV/AIDS and to push for increased funding and research dedicated to finding cures and treatments.

Supportive figures in her life played a crucial role in her ascent to scientific prominence. Mentors and colleagues who recognized her potential provided guidance and opportunities that were pivotal in her career. Such support networks are invaluable, offering encouragement and resources that enable individuals to thrive in competitive environments.

Flossie Wong-Staal defied societal norms to pursue her dreams and her bold decision to continue her education in the United States. Her relentless curiosity sparked a lifelong quest for knowledge that guided her from UCLA to becoming a trailblazer in HIV/AIDS research.

Working with this virus is like putting your hand in a treasure chest. Every time you put your hand in, you pull out a gem. –Flossie Wong-Staal

You're the One to Change the World

What's your biggest dream? If you had a superpower, what would it be? Imagine you found Aladdin's lamp and the genie asked you, "What would you like to change in the world?" Do you know what your answer would be?

All the women you've just read about had dreams, just like you. But guess what? No genie came up to offer them three wishes, and they didn't get any superhuman gifts. Fortunately, they found out early that the true magic lay inside themselves. They had the power to break down any barrier and pursue their dreams. Now, it's your turn to light up the strength within you and choose your path to make the world a better place.

Have you ever heard about vision boards? They're a wonderful visual tool that make your ideas come to life through images. We're going to create a vision board of who you want to be to change the world.

First, take a pen and a sheet of paper, or open your favorite writing tool on your device. Create a list of all the amazing things you are. Then, think about what you would like to be to make a change in the world and leave an enduring footprint.

Write down your name and use each letter of it to name a quality that makes you unique. Here you have an example using my name!

Playful

crEative

Grateful

Generous

joYful

Then, turn them into what you want to achieve. Like this...

- I'm playful, so when I grow up, I'll be exploratory and discover new things.
- I'm creative, so I'll come up with innovative ideas.
- I'm grateful, so I'll follow these great women's steps.
- I'm generous, so I'll contribute to spreading interest in science.
- I'm joyful, so my ideas will bring hope and happiness to everyone.

Now, look up pictures or photos that you relate to those thoughts and make a collage. You can also draw letters or cut them out from magazines and write your words of power.

Look at yourself in the mirror and say these words to yourself. They are part of what you are, and they hold the secret formula to unfold the magic and power that lies inside you.

The world is waiting; go for it!

Conclusion

In the stories of these remarkable women, you've found more than just tales of overcoming hurdles—you've discovered a testament to the power of resilience and determination in the face of adversity. These pioneering women in medicine stood against societal norms and personal challenges, showing us that persistence can indeed break barriers and pave the way for transformative changes.

Throughout history, the women in this book have shown how crucial it is to build networks of support and mentorship. They remind us that while individual effort is vital, the power of collective strength can elevate ambitions to new heights. Susan La Flesche Picotte serves as a shining example. With her community's backing, she became the first Native American woman to earn a medical degree, and also addressed healthcare disparities head-on. Together with her community, she established the first hospital on a reservation, showcasing how local support can create waves of positive change in healthcare outcomes.

Education opens doors and creates pathways for self-advancement and the upliftment of entire communities. Many of these extraordinary women realized that their knowledge had the power to educate others, ensuring that future generations could benefit from their experiences and insights. Mary Breckinridge, through her founding of the Frontier Nursing Service, exemplifies this legacy. Her vision brought about educational initiatives that drastically improved healthcare delivery in rural Appalachia, highlighting the profound impact education can have on nurturing innovation and progress.

Advocacy runs like a lifeline through the stories of these women. Their relentless dedication to public health and patient safety made lasting impressions on healthcare systems worldwide, ensuring better standards of care and protection for generations to come.

As a young girl with dreams of venturing into medicine, there's so much to take away from these stories. As you learn about history, you're connecting with mentors whose stories mirror the possibilities within your own life. These women were once where you are now: searching for direction, questioning their paths, and daring to dream beyond their immediate horizons. They've proved that it's possible to carve out a niche in fields traditionally dominated by others, using their voices to make powerful statements of change and progress.

Think of every obstacle as a stepping stone, each one a chance to prove your mettle and expand your capabilities. As you flip through the pages of your own life, remember that setbacks and failures aren't endpoints but rather chapters in a larger story—an opportunity for growth and learning. The path may not always be clear, but with persistence, courage, and a sense of community, you can achieve anything you set your mind to.

Let this book serve as an invitation to explore your potential and a challenge to break your own barriers. Imagine the impact you could make if you chose to follow in the footsteps of these pioneers, or perhaps to blaze entirely new trails of your own. Whether it's through small acts of kindness, volunteering, pursuing your studies with vigor, or simply supporting your peers, your contributions matter more than you know.

Always keep in mind that success isn't merely an individual journey. Look around you at your friends, family, and educators, and draw strength from them. Build and cherish a network of allies who believe in your dreams and are committed to seeing you thrive. When we work together, pooling our resources and strengths, we become unstoppable forces for good and agents of change.

Finally, let curiosity and compassion guide you. The medical and scientific world is ever-evolving, with endless opportunities for discovery and advancement. By staying curious, you ensure that you're always learning, adapting, and growing. And by remaining compassionate, you guarantee that your efforts will be rooted in a desire to improve lives and uplift those around you.

In closing, may you carry forward the torch of these exceptional women, lighting the way for yourself and others. Let their achievements inspire you to seek out your passions with confidence and boldness. Remember, the most significant breakthroughs often begin with a single step toward the unknown. Embrace your journey with optimism and enthusiasm, knowing that, like the women before you, your dreams possess the power to change the world.

References

Alexander, K. L., & Rothberg, E. (2023). *Mary Edwards Walker.* National Women's History Museum. https://www.womenshistory.org/education-resources/biographies/mary-edwards-walker

American Chemical Society. (n.d.). *Gertrude Elion (1918–1999).* https://www.acs.org/education/whatischemistry/women-scientists/gertrude-elion.html

Apgar score. (n.d.). MedlinePlus. https://medlineplus.gov/ency/article/003402.htm

Apgar, V. (n.d.). Quote. In National Women's Hall of Fame. (n.d.). *Dr. Virginia Apgar: The woman behind the Apgar Score.* Google Arts & Culture. https://artsandculture.google.com/story/dr-virginia-apgar-the-woman-behind-the-apgar-score-national-women-s-hall-of-fame/xgVxylfnmvRdLA?hl=en

Aravind, M., & Chung, K. C. (2010). Evidence-based medicine and hospital reform: Tracing origins back to Florence Nightingale.

Plastic and Reconstructive Surgery, 125(1), 403-409. https://doi.org/10.1097/prs.0b013e3181c2bb89

Barbara McClintock. (n.d.). The Nobel Prize. https://www.nobelprize.org/womenwhochangedscience/stories/barbara-mcclintock

Barbara McClintock: Jumping gene pioneer—perseverance in face of skepticism. (n.d.). Editverse. https://editverse.com/barbara-mcclintock-transposons-scientific-skepticism/

Bath, P. (n.d.). Quote. In Davidson, M. (2005, March 3). *Innovative lives: The right to sight: Patricia Bath.* The Lemelson Center for the Study of Invention and Innovation. https://invention.si.edu/invention-stories/innovative-lives-right-sight-patricia-bath

Blackwell, E. (n.d.). *Elizabeth Blackwell quote.* BrainyQuote. https://www.brainyquote.com/quotes/elizabeth_blackwell_317643

Boehm, J. S., & Jacks, T. (2024). Radical collaboration: Reimagining cancer team science. *Cancer Discovery, 14*(4), 563–568. https://doi.org/10.1158/2159-8290.cd-23-1496

Breckinridge, M. (n.d.). Quote. In Frontier Nursing University. (2016, January 26). *One of our favorite quotes from Mary Breckinridge, founder of Frontier Nursing University* [Image attached] [Post]. Facebook.

https://www.facebook.com/FrontierSchool/photos/one-of-our-favorite-quotes/10154029964573394/

Burgess, A. (2017, September 27). *The unconventional life of Mary Walker, the only woman to have received the U.S. Medal of Honor.* Atlas Obscura. https://www.atlasobscura.com/articles/mary-walker-feminist-dress-reform-equal-rights

Cartwright, R. L. (2012, November 27). *Sister Kenny Institute revolutionized treatment of polio patients.* MinnPost. https://www.minnpost.com/mnopedia/2012/11/sister-kenny-institute-revolutionized-treatment-polio-patients/

Centers for Disease Control and Prevention. (2024, May 16). *Tribal contributions to public health.* https://www.cdc.gov/tribal-health/tribal-stories/index.html

Clarke, A. & Martin, J. H. (2023). *A*nne Laura Dorinthea McLaren DBE. 26 April 1927—7 July 2007. *Biographical Memoirs of Fellows of the Royal Society. Royal Society*, *74*, 309–337. http://doi.org/10.1098/rsbm.2022.0053

Concorde Staff. (2022, October 27). Native Americans who impacted the healthcare industry. *Concorde.* https://www.concorde.edu/blog/native-americans-who-impacted-healthcare-industry

Dammann, N. (1980). The Frontier nursing service as an agent of change. *Walden Dissertations and Doctoral Studies*, 250. https://scholarworks.waldenu.edu/dissertations/250/

Davidson, M. (2005, March 3). *Innovative lives: The right to sight: Patricia Bath.* The Lemelson Center for the Study of Invention and Innovation. https://invention.si.edu/invention-stories/innovative-lives-right-sight-patricia-bath

Delaine, T. (2020, March 6). *Anne McLaren: Pioneer of embryology and IVF technology.* Pretty Smart Science.

https://prettysmartscience.com/2020/03/06/anne-mclaren-pioneer-of-embryology-and-ivf-technology/

Dr. Patricia E. Bath. (2015, June 3). Changing the Face of Medicine. https://cfmedicine.nlm.nih.gov/physicians/biography_26.html

Dreier, P. (2015, August 10). *Frances Kelsey: The government bureaucrat who may have saved your life.* The American Prospect. https://prospect.org/environment/frances-kelsey-government-bureaucrat-may-saved-life/

Elion, G. B. (n.d.). *Gertrude B. Elion quote.* BrainyQuote. https://www.brainyquote.com/quotes/gertrude_b_elion_728592

Elliott, E. (2016, November 30). Women in Science: Jane C. Wright revolutionized cancer research (1919–2013). *The Jackson Laboratory.* https://www.jax.org/news-and-insights/jax-blog/2016/november/women-in-science-jane-wright

Elliott, E. (2017, October 11). Women in Science: Helen Taussig (1898–1986). *The Jackson Laboratory.* https://www.jax.org/news-and-insights/jax-blog/2017/october/women-in-science-helen-taussig

Estel, C. M. (2021, March 19). *Dr. Mary Edwards Walker: A pioneer for women's rights.* The Progressive Magazine.

https://progressive.org/latest/mary-edwards-walker-estel-210319/

Falzone, L., Salomone, S., & Libra, M. (2018, November 12). Evolution of cancer pharmacological treatments at the turn of the third millennium. *Frontiers in Pharmacology, 9.* https://doi.org/10.3389/fphar.2018.01300

Fee, E., & Garofalo, M. E. (2010). Florence Nightingale and the Crimean War. *American Journal of Public Health*, *100*, 1591. https://doi.org/10.2105/ajph.2009.188607

Fielding, S. (2022, February 22). Overlooked no more: Mary Eliza Mahoney, who opened doors in nursing. *The New York Times.* https://www.nytimes.com/2022/02/19/obituaries/mary-eliza-mahoney-overlooked.html

The first American Indian doctor. (n.d.). American Masters. https://www.pbs.org/wnet/americanmasters/meet-first-american-indian-woman-physician-ienwy3/14818/

Flam, F. (2020, July 20). Flossie Wong-Staal, who unlocked mystery of H.I.V., dies at 73. *The New York Times.*

https://www.nytimes.com/2020/07/17/science/flossie-wong-staal-who-unlocked-mystery-of-hiv-dies-at-73.html

4th medical trip of American facial plastic reconstructive surgeons. (2024, December 12). Razom. https://www.razomforukraine.org/category/project-activity/education/?k=31-561-1

Frances Oldham Kelsey: Medical reviewer famous for averting a public health tragedy. (2018, February 1). U.S. Food and Drug Administration. https://www.fda.gov/about-fda/fda-history-exhibits/frances-oldham-kelsey-medical-reviewer-famous-averting-public-health-tragedy

Gertrude B. Elion. (n.d.). The Nobel Prize. https://www.nobelprize.org/womenwhochangedscience/stories/gertrude-elion

Godlewski, N. (2018, June 7). *Doctor Virginia Apgar quotes: Creator of Apgar Scale honored with Google Doodle.* Newsweek. https://www.newsweek.com/virginia-apgar-quotes-doctor-apgar-scale-said-dr-google-doodle-964305

Gulley T. (2022). Review of: *Wide neighborhoods: A story of the frontier nursing service. Journal of Appalachian Health*, *4*(1), 61–64. https://doi.org/10.13023/jah.0401.07

Guy's and St Thomas' NHS Foundation Trust. (n.d.). *The Nightingale training school and home for nurses.*

https://guysandstthomas.shorthandstories.com/the-nightingale-training-school/index.html

Headrick, A., Qureshi, A. M., Ghanayem, N. S., Heinle, J. S., & Anders, M. (2022, July). In-hospital morbidity and mortality after modified Blalock-Taussig-Thomas Shunts. *The Annals of Thoracic Surgery, 114*(1), 168-175. https://doi.org/10.1016/j.athoracsur.2021.11.003

Hernandez, M. A., Sharma, R., Xu, Y., & Feinstein, E. (2024). A genetic key lay hidden in the shores of Lake Maracaibo—Historical review of genetic research of Huntington's disease in US and Venezuela (P1-1.015). *Neurology, 102*(17 Suppl 1). https://doi.org/10.1212/wnl.0000000000205982

Iheduru-Anderson, K., Okoro, F. O. & Moore, S. S. (2022). Diversity and inclusion or tokens? A qualitative study of Black women academic nurse leaders in the United States. *Global Qualitative Nursing Research, 9*. https://doi.org/10.1177/23333936211073116

International Parkinson and Movement Disorder Society. (2023, January 9). History of movement disorders: Huntington disease in Venezuela [Audio podcast episode]. In *MDS Podcast.* International Parkinson and Movement Disorder Society. https://www.movementdisorders.org/Podcasts/History-of-Movement-Disorders--Huntington-Disease-in-Venezuela.htm

Kays, H. (2022, April 4). *Breaking barriers: A history of Mary Eliza Mahoney.* American Association of Nurse Practitioners.

https://www.aanp.org/news-feed/breaking-barriers-a-history-of-mary-eliza-mahoney

Kelsey, F. O. (n.d.). Quote. In Benderly, B. L. (2015, August 12). *A legacy of drug safety.* Science. https://www.science.org/content/article/legacy-drug-safety

Kenny, E. (n.d.). *Elizabeth Kenny quote.* BrainyQuote. https://www.brainyquote.com/quotes/elizabeth_kenny_729966

Kenyon, G. (2020). Flossie Wong-Staal. *The Lancet Infectious Diseases, 20*(9), 1022. https://doi.org/10.1016/S1473-3099(20)30645-9

La Flesche, S. (n.d.). Quote. In Peone, C. (2020, July 20). *Susan La Flesche Picotte: A woman trailblazer.* Carmen Peone. https://carmenpeone.com/susan-la-flesche-picotte-a-woman-trailblazer/

Lacor Hospital Annual Workshop. (2014, June 25). *Social Promise.* https://socialpromiseblog.wordpress.com/category/lacor-hospital/page/2/

Lady Science. (2018, November 15). *Dr. Jane C. Wright and the making of modern oncology.* The New Inquiry. https://thenewinquiry.com/blog/dr-jane-c-wright-and-the-making-of-modern-oncology/

Lasker, M. (n.d.). Quote. In National Institutes of Health. (2007, June 21). *Papers of medical philanthropist and NIH benefactor Mary Lasker added to the National Library of Medicine's profiles in science web site.* https://www.nih.gov/news-events/news-releases/papers-medical-philanthropist-nih-benefactor-mary-lasker-added-national-library-medicines-profiles-science-web-site

Lee, W. (2024). A critical multicultural analysis of underrepresented figures in contemporary STEM picture-book biographies for children (2020–2022). *Multicultural Perspectives, 26*(1), 37-58. https://doi.org/10.1080/15210960.2024.2350074

Legendarywomen. (2016, August 15). *Remembering Frances Oldham Kelsey: How one woman prevented an American tragedy*. Medium. https://medium.com/legendary-women/remembering-frances-oldham-kelsey-how-one-woman-prevented-an-american-tragedy-9c90147ea6c1

Levy, B. (2023, October 30). New Lasker scholars are coming for cancer. *I Am Intramural.* https://irp.nih.gov/blog/post/2023/10/new-lasker-scholars-are-coming-for-cancer

Liao, S., Lavender, C., & Zhai, H. (2024). Factors influencing the research impact in cancer research: A collaboration and knowledge network analysis. *Health Research Policy and Systems, 22*, 96. https://doi.org/10.1186/s12961-024-01205-8

Lim, G., Facco, F. L., Nathan, N., Waters, J. H., Wong, C. A., & Eltzschig, H. K. (2018). A review of the impact of obstetric anesthesia on maternal and neonatal outcomes. *Anesthesiology, 129*(1), 192-215. https://doi.org/10.1097/aln.0000000000002182

Liu, W., & Liu, Y. (2016). Youyou Tu: Significance of winning the 2015 Nobel Prize in Physiology or Medicine. *Cardiovascular Diagnosis and Therapy, 6*(1). https://doi.org/10.3978/j.issn.2223-3652.2015.12.11

Lodge, Z. (2024, June 18). Speeding past barriers: McLaren's 60 scholars initiative returns to boost women in STEM, motorsports. *International Business Times.* https://www.ibtimes.co.uk/speeding-past-barriers-mclarens-60-scholars-initiative-returns-boost-women-stem-motorsports-1724986

Mahoney, M. E. (n.d.). Quote. In Fielding, S. (2022, February 22). Overlooked no more: Mary Eliza Mahoney, who opened doors in nursing. *The New York Times.* https://www.nytimes.com/2022/02/19/obituaries/mary-eliza-mahoney-overlooked.html

Malaria is once again killing in Uganda. (2015, July 7). *Social Promise.* https://socialpromiseblog.wordpress.com/tag/gulu/page/2/

Mary Breckinridge. (n.d.). National Women's Hall of Fame. https://www.womenofthehall.org/inductee/mary-breckinridge/

Mattison, M. (2022, February 9). *A celebration of 14 famous Black nurses in history.* Chamberlain University. https://www.chamberlain.edu/blog/a-celebration-of-10-famous-black-nurses-in-history

McClintock, B. (n.d.-a). *Barbara McClintock quote.* BrainyQuote. https://www.brainyquote.com/quotes/barbara_mcclintock_390227

McClintock, B. (n.d.-b). *Barbara McClintock quote.* BrainyQuote. https://www.brainyquote.com/authors/barbara-mcclintock-quotes

McLaren, A. L. D. (n.d.). Quote. In Clarke, A. & Martin, J. H. (2023). Anne Laura Dorinthea McLaren DBE. 26 April 1927—7 July 2007. *Biographical Memoirs of Fellows of the Royal Society. Royal Society, 74*, 309–337. http://doi.org/10.1098/rsbm.2022.0053

Memorial Sloan Kettering Cancer Center. (n.d.). *The life and legacy of Gertrude Elion.* https://www.mskcc.org/research-advantage/

marie-josee-kravis-women-science-endeavor-wise/wise-symposia/life-and-legacy-gertrude-elion

Michals, D. (2015). *Elizabeth Blackwell.* National Women's History Museum. https://www.womenshistory.org/education-resources/biographies/elizabeth-blackwell

Morantz-Sanchez, R. (1992) Feminist theory and historical practice: Rereading Elizabeth Blackwell. *History and Theory 31*(4), 51–69. https://doi.org/10.2307/2505415

Nallamotu, S., Vankayalapati, A., & Paruchuri, S. (2024). Dr. Elizabeth Blackwell (1821–1910): Opening doors to women in medicine. *Cureus, 16*(10), e71899. https://doi.org/10.7759/cureus.71899

National Institutes of Health. (2007, June 21). *Papers of medical philanthropist and NIH benefactor Mary Lasker added to the National Library of Medicine's profiles in science web site.* https://www.nih.gov/news-events/news-releases/papers-medical-philanthropist-nih-benefactor-mary-lasker-added-national-library-medicines-profiles-science-web-site

National Park Service. (n.d.). *Dr. Mary Edwards Walker.* https://www.nps.gov/people/mary-walker.htm

National Women's Hall of Fame. (n.d.-a). *Virginia Apgar.* https://www.womenofthehall.org/inductee/virginia-apgar/

National Women's Hall of Fame. (n.d.-b). *Dr. Virginia Apgar: The woman behind the Apgar Score.* Google Arts & Culture. https://artsandculture.google.com/story/dr-virginia-apgar-the-woman-behind-the-apgar-score-national-women-s-hall-of-fame/xgVxylfnmvRdLA?hl=en

Nightingale, F. (n.d.). *Florence Nightingale quote.* Brainy Quote. https://www.brainyquote.com/quotes/florence_nightingale_752504

Nocco, M. A., McGill, B. M., MacKenzie, C. M., Tonietto, R. K., Dudney, J., Bletz, M. C., Young, T., & Kuebbing, S. E. (2021). Mentorship, equity, and research productivity: Lessons from a pandemic. *Biological Conservation, 225*, 108966,. https://doi.org/10.1016/j.biocon.2021.108966

oliviaoconnor182. (2025, January 23). *Ethical dilemmas in medical research and treatment.* Quizlet. https://quizlet.com/study-guides/ethical-dilemmas-in-medical-research-and-treatment-52419ee4-1d09-4024-9ab9-b64df7c3b71c

Paik, S. J., Choe, S. M. M., Otto, W. J., & Rahman, Z. (2018, April 5). Learning about the lives and early experiences of notable Asian American women: Productive giftedness, childhood traits, and supportive conditions. *Journal for the Education of the Gifted, 41*(2), 160–192. https://doi.org/10.1177/0162353218763927

Peone, C. (2020, July 20). *Susan La Flesche Picotte: A woman trailblazer.* Carmen Peone. https://carmenpeone.com/susan-la-flesche-picotte-a-woman-trailblazer/

Ravindran, S. (2012). Barbara McClintock and the discovery of jumping genes. *Proceedings of the National Academy of Sciences,*

109(50), 20198-20199 https://doi.org/10.1073/pnas.1219372109

Ray, A. R., Haines, D., & Grell, R. (2024, May 26). Virginia Apgar (1909-1974): The Mother of Neonatal Resuscitation. *Cureus, 16(5).* https://doi.org/10.7759/cureus.61115

Roberts, J. S., Patterson, A. K., & Uhlmann, W. R. (2020). Genetic testing for neurodegenerative diseases: Ethical and health communication challenges. *Neurobiology of Disease, 141*, 104871,. https://doi.org/10.1016/j.nbd.2020.104871

Rogers, K. (2024, November 26). Elizabeth Kenny. In *Encyclopedia Britannica.* https://www.britannica.com/biography/Elizabeth-Kenny

Rogers, N. (2014, May 22). *Polio wars: Sister Kenny and the golden age of American medicine* [Book review]. Oxford Academic. https://doi.org/10.1093/acprof:oso/9780195380590.001.0001

The Royal Society. (n.d.). *The road to IVF: Dame Anne McLaren.* Google Arts & Culture. https://artsandculture.google.com/story/the-road-to-ivf-dame-anne-mclaren-the-royal-society/JwWB6bxH9vTk2A?hl=en

Shampo, M. A., & Kyle, R. A. (1999). Mary Breckinridge—Pioneer nurse brings modern nursing to rural environment. *Mayo Clinic Proceedings, 74*(12), 1312. https://doi.org/10.4065/74.12.1312

StemBot. (2022, May 3). *Celebrating Asian Heritage & STEM.* STEM Minds. https://www.stemminds.com/asian-heritage-month/

Susan La Flesche Picotte: A pathbreaking doctor from Indigenous America. (2021, March 11). Local Initiatives Support Corporation. https://www.lisc.org/our-stories/story/susan-la-flesche-picotte-pathbreaking-doctor-indigenous-america/

Taussig, H. B. (n.d.). Quote. In Concepts. (2024, November). *Here's an inspirational quote from Dr. Helen Brooke Taussig.* [Image attached] [Post]. LinkedIn. https://www.linkedin.com/posts/comcepts_heres-an-inspirational-quote-from-dr-helen-activity-7257142682127331328-3YeH

Teasdale-Corti, L. (n.d.). Quote. In Canadian Museum for Human Rights. (2017, December 14). *Have you heard of Dr. Lucille Teasdale Corti?* [Image attached] [Post]. Facebook. https://www.facebook.com/canadianmuseumforhumanrights/

posts/have-you-heard-of-dr-lucille-teasdale-corti-she-was-one-of-canadas-first-female-/10156074983825513/?_rdc=2&_rdr

10 women who've transformed healthcare in Australia. (n.d.). GPEx. https://gpex.com.au/news/10-women-whove-transformed-healthcare-in-australia/

Thakur, J., Choudhari, S. G., & Gaidhane, A. (2024). Pioneering physician: Dr. Elizabeth Blackwell and the path to medical history. *Cureus, 16*(9), e68713. https://doi.org/10.7759/cureus.68713

The Thalidomide Trust. (n.d.). *About thalidomide.* (n.d.). The Thalidomide Trust. https://www.thalidomidetrust.org/about-us/about-thalidomide/

Treisman, R. (2021, September 27). *Meet the first 2 Black women to be inducted into the National Inventors Hall of Fame.* NPR. https://www.npr.org/2021/09/27/1040795026/patricia-bath-marian-croak-national-inventors-hall-of-fame-first-black-women

Tu Youyou. (n.d.). The Nobel Prize. https://www.nobelprize.org/womenwhochangedscience/stories/tu-youyou

Uhlmann, W. R. (2010). Book review: The woman who walked into the sea: Huntington's and the making of a genetic disease. *The*

American Journal of Human Genetics, 86(6), 830-831. http://dx.doi.org/10.1016/j.ajhg.2010.05.007

Waggoner, M. R., & Lyerly, A. D. (2022). Clinical trials in pregnancy and the "shadows of thalidomide": Revisiting the legacy of Frances Kelsey. *Contemporary Clinical Trials, 119*, 106806. https://doi.org/10.1016/j.cct.2022.106806

Walker, M. E. (n.d.). Quote. In Whitman-Walker. (n.d.). *Meet Dr. Mary Edwards "Walker."* https://www.whitman-walker.org/meet-dr-mary-edwards-walker

Wexler, N. (n.d.). Quote. In Uhlmann, W. R. (2010). Book review: The woman who walked into the sea: Huntington's and the making of a genetic disease. *The American Journal of Human Genetics, 86*(6), 830-831. http://dx.doi.org/10.1016/j.ajhg.2010.05.007

Whitman-Walker. (n.d.). *Meet Dr. Mary Edwards "Walker."* https://www.whitman-walker.org/meet-dr-mary-edwards-walker

Williamson, L. (2024, March 28). *Dr. Helen Taussig's work saved "blue babies" and made her the mother of pediatric cardiology.* American Heart

Association. https://www.heart.org/en/news/2024/03/28/dr-helen-taussigs-work-saved-blue-babies

Winkfield, D. K. (2021, February 17). *Dr. Patricia Bath: Bringing vision to community health.* Dr. Karen Winkfield. https://www.drkarenwinkfield.com/post/dr-patricia-bath

Wisconsin Center for Nursing. (n.d.). *Mary Elizabeth Mahoney – First African-American nurse.* https://wicenterfornursing.org/mary-elizabeth-mahoney-first-african-american-nurse/

Women in Medicine Legacy Foundation. (2020, March 17). *Helen B. Taussig, MD: A pioneer in the diagnosis and treatment of congenital heart disease.* https://www.wimlf.org/blog/helen-b-taussig-md

Women's history month—Barbara McClintock. (2014, March 1). Cold Spring Harbor Laboratory. https://www.cshl.edu/archives-blog/womens-history-month-barbara-mcclintock/

Wong-Staal, F. (n.d.). In Flam, F. (2020, July 20). Flossie Wong-Staal, who unlocked mystery of H.I.V., dies at 73. *The New York Times.*

https://www.nytimes.com/2020/07/17/science/flossie-wong-staal-who-unlocked-mystery-of-hiv-dies-at-73.html

Wright, J. C. (n.d.). Quote. In *Quotes by Jane Cook Wright.* (n.d.). POC Quotes. https://poc.nestagarrick.com/authors/jane-cooke-wright/

Youyou, T. (n.d.). Quote. In *TuYouyou quotes.* (n.d.) What Should I Read Next? https://www.whatshouldireadnext.com/quotes/tu-youyou-when-you-are-entrusted-with

Made in the USA
Monee, IL
13 September 2026

62981870R00075